Pharmacology
for respiratory therapists

Pharmacology for respiratory therapists

Hugh S. Mathewson, M.D.

Professor of Anesthesiology and
Medical Director, Respiratory Therapy,
The University of Kansas Medical Center,
College of Health Sciences and Hospital,
Kansas City, Kansas

The C. V. Mosby Company

Saint Louis   1977

Library of Congress Cataloging in Publication Data

Mathewson, Hugh S
    Pharmacology for respiratory therapists.

    Includes bibliographical references and index.
    1. Pharmacology. 2. Inhalation therapy.
I. Title. [DNLM: 1. Pharmacology.
2. Inhalation therapy. QV4 M429p]
RM300.M197   615'.64   76-41196
ISBN 0-8016-3160-2

GW/M/M 9 8 7 6 5 4 3 2 1

To
**Geoff, Brian,
Cathy,** and **Jenny**

Preface

The education of the respiratory therapist must include many facets of pharmacology. The properties of oxygen and of drugs to be given by aerosol are most obvious; the therapist will administer oxygen and drugs at times with little or no supervision. Most bronchoactive drugs have potent cardiovascular side effects and these must be anticipated if catastrophe is to be avoided. Emphasis is placed on beta adrenergic agents, which have great potential for harm if used injudiciously. Other sections of the text deal with substances that lyse secretions, drugs given to facilitate respiratory assistance or control, and antimicrobials.

An introductory chapter initiates the student to the basic terms and concepts of pharmacology. Some important but difficult topics, such as structure-activity relations and neurohumoral transmission, are treated cursorily; brevity is dictated by appropriateness of need. After the sections on bronchodilator and mucokinetic agents, muscle relaxant, local anesthetic, and central depressant drugs are considered with respect to their applications in respiratory care. Oxygen and other therapeutic gases occupy the ensuing pages, and finally a chapter on antimicrobial therapy is presented.

It is hoped that this brief text can be encompassed by the student in the time allocated to pharmacology in the respiratory therapy curriculum. Larger reference sources are cited for further study. I shall be most satisfied if students are motivated to further reading beyond this review, to achieve the comprehension in depth so essential to the development of sound clinical judgment.

I wish to express thanks for support and encouragement to my ARRT colleagues, David C. Assmann, Gareth B. Gish, and

Joan P. Taylor, and to Kasumi Arakawa, M.D., Acting Chairman of Anesthesiology at the University of Kansas Medical Center. Finally, a word of praise for her untiring efforts to Peggy Zacher, who converted illegible notes into an accurate and artistic manuscript.

Hugh S. Mathewson

Contents

Contents

1 Basic pharmacology

Pharmacology is the basic discipline concerning the actions of drugs. This monograph will be concerned only with the knowledge appropriate to problems in man, or *clinical pharmacology*. Included are the applications of drugs to the treatment of disease; this is termed *therapeutics*.

The respiratory therapist must be acquainted with the actions and uses of many therapeutic substances. A number of them are given by inhalation (e.g., oxygen, carbon dioxide, helium, nitrogen). Also solutions of drugs can be delivered to the bronchial tree as aerosols. Bronchodilators, mucolytic agents, corticosteroids, and antibiotics comprise most of these. In addition, the therapist must be familiar with drugs administered by other routes that affect respiratory function.

Routes of administration of drugs

To produce a systemic therapeutic effect, a drug must gain access to the circulation to be transported to its site of action. In ambulatory patients this is ordinarily accomplished by oral administration of the drug, which then is absorbed from the gastrointestinal tract. A similar mode of entry is *rectal* administration.

Some drugs cannot be given via the gastrointestinal tract because decomposition or inactivation occurs. In such instances, they must be given *parenterally* (i.e., by injection). A solution of the drug is introduced into the subcutaneous tissue or muscle or, if rapid onset of action is desired, directly into the circulating blood. The latter route, termed *intravenous* when a vein is entered, is the preferable mode of administration in clinical emergencies.

Application of a drug, either solid or liquid, to the skin or a mucous surface is known as *topical* administration. Local anesthetic drugs may be employed in this manner to facilitate instrumentation of the airway, such as intubation and bronchoscopy. Aerosolized solutions of bronchoactive drugs may be introduced into the tracheobronchial tree. Direct instillation of the solution into the airway is occasionally required for mucolysis and removal of secretions.

Inhalation is the route employed for administration of gases, which are absorbed into the circulation via the bronchial mucosa and the alveolocapillary membrane. Therapeutic gases include oxygen, carbon dioxide, and helium. Inhalation anesthetic agents include gases and the vapors of volatile liquids.

The basic advantages and disadvantages of the common routes of administration are summarized in Table 1-1.

Table 1-1. Routes of administration of drugs

	Advantages	*Disadvantages*
Oral (or rectal)	Convenience, economy	Absorption may be variable and erratic; requires patient cooperation
Subcutaneous	Ease of administration; rapid absorption of aqueous solutions	Only limited volumes of solution can be given; irritating solutions may cause sloughs
Intramuscular	Ease of administration; more rapid absorption than subcutaneous route	Unsuitable if patient is on anticoagulants
Intravenous	Immediate action permits titration of dosage; large volumes can be given; irritating substances may be administered if well diluted	Increased risk of overdose or untoward side effects; occasional difficulty of venipuncture
Inhalation Topical administration of aerosols	Immediate action permits titration of dosage; direct delivery to site of action	Requires special equipment; risk of overdose or untoward side effects; requires patient cooperation

Principal and side effects of drugs

The classification of drugs in pharmacology is based on the principal therapeutic action exhibited by each drug. Thus a local anesthetic, such as lidocaine, is described in company with other compounds having similar action. Most drugs possess a single therapeutic action; others may have many. Usually, however, a single mode of action will account for more than one therapeutic effect. Lidocaine may be used to suppress cardiac arrhythmia, but the effect on the myocardial conduction tissue is probably the same as on ordinary nerve fibers. Isoproterenol, often employed as a bronchodilator, is also a powerful cardiac stimulant. These actions are explained by the assumption that similar receptor cells are activated on both bronchiolar smooth muscle and myocardium.

Even with ordinary doses, nearly all drugs will show other effects beside the desired therapeutic action. These are termed *side actions*. Often they are responsible for unwanted symptoms that may limit the usefulness of the drug. Isoproterenol is useful in acute asthma; but its cardiac action, resulting in increased work of the heart and acceleration of the rate, may militate against its application in the patient with heart disease.

Mode of action of drugs

Drugs are substances exerting special actions on physiologic functions; these actions, properly applied, have therapeutic value. The selectivity of drugs suggests an affinity for a cellular site, which in turn connotes a peculiarity of chemical structure enabling the drug molecule to fit or penetrate a complementary configuration on the cell surface. The assumption that some type of reversible bonding occurs between a drug and its cellular receptor site forms the basis of our concepts regarding the mechanisms of drug action.

Potency and efficacy

The more selective the affinity of a drug for a special receptor site, the more *potent* it is likely to be (i.e., the smaller the dose required to elicit the desired response). The potencies of comparable drugs may be defined as the doses which produce the same effect, as measured by a given test. Some drugs are more powerful than others, however, and will show higher magnitudes of activity. This property is referred to as *efficacy* and can be viewed as the "ceiling" of the drug effect. Thus two drugs of the same class may have differing potencies, or different therapeutic doses; and, in addition, one may be more efficacious (i.e., capable of exerting a greater maximum activity).

Structure-activity relations

The molecular structure needed to elicit a given drug action is of primary importance and is the most rational way to identify a drug as belonging to a certain class. Understanding molecular structure requires some foreknowledge of the form and language of chemistry. The structural formula is a conventional representation of a three-dimensional molecule; the student of pharmacology must be able to recognize the molecular characteristics that identify the various classes of drugs.

Chemical formulas. A few words may be interposed concerning the conventional depiction of organic compounds. Bonds connecting the atoms of simple groups or radicals (e.g., CH_3, CO, NH_2) are ordinarily not shown. Ring structures are often denoted by polygons, each corner of the polygon representing a carbon atom with its substituent hydrogens. Thus cyclohex-

ane, $CH_2 \begin{smallmatrix} CH_2—CH_2 \\ \\ CH_2—CH_2 \end{smallmatrix} CH_2$, may be shown as ⬡. Any element other

than hydrogen attached to a ring carbon must be so indicated;

for example, monochlorocyclohexane is ⬡—Cl.

If the ring contains elements other than carbon (heterocyclic), the polygon is always broken at the position of a noncarbon atom.

For example, piperidine, $\begin{smallmatrix} CH_2 \\ CH_2 \quad CH_2 \\ CH_2 \quad CH_2 \\ N \\ H \end{smallmatrix}$ becomes ⬡$\begin{smallmatrix} \\ N \\ H \end{smallmatrix}$

Many ring structures contain doubly bonded carbons; frequently the double bonds alternate with single bonds, in a manner exemplified by benzene: $\underset{\underset{\displaystyle CH}{CH\diagdown_{\diagup}CH}}{\overset{\overset{\displaystyle CH}{CH\diagup^{\diagdown}CH}}{\|\quad\|}}$. This often is written

as [benzene ring structure] ; however, the bonds oscillate and the form [benzene ring structure] is

equally correct. In recent years the noncommittal form [benzene ring with circle] has been more widely accepted.

Nature of drug-receptor union. Early workers in pharmacology (Langley, Ehrlich, E. Fischer) postulated the existence of a cellular receptor into which the drug molecule fits, similar to the way a key fits into a lock. This simplistic model has been revised and extended until it now appears to be a specialized version of the enzyme-substrate complex. The ability of a compound to form such a complex depends on the molecular structure of the compound; thus drugs of similar structure might be expected to show similarity of pharmacologic action.

Certain identifiable chemical groupings are essential to drug-receptor union and appear consistently in drugs exhibiting the same effects. Fig. 1 shows the chemical groups that confer bronchodilator (beta$_2$ adrenergic) activity in epinephrine, isoproterenol, and terbutaline. Bronchodilator activity is accentuated as the terminal nitrogen is "loaded" with more hydrocarbon groupings and may be assumed to improve the drug-receptor fit.

To meet the specifications of the receptor cell, the spatial arrangement of the active groups must follow definite dimensional requirements and the union must result in discharge of the receptor cell, whether muscle or glandular in nature. A compound that exhibits both affinity and efficacy is termed an *agonist*. By contrast, a similar compound may be identified that fits the receptor but elicits no response, in other words, possesses affinity but no efficacy. By occupying receptor sites, it can pre-

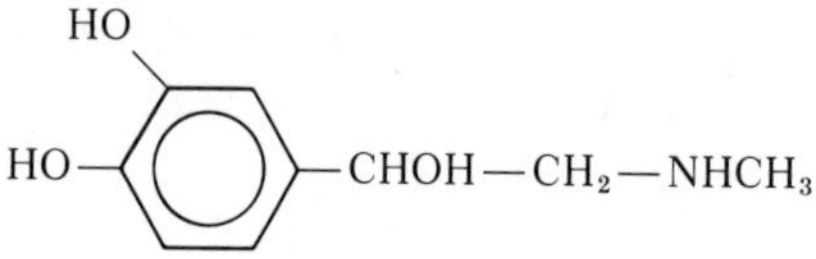

Epinephrine

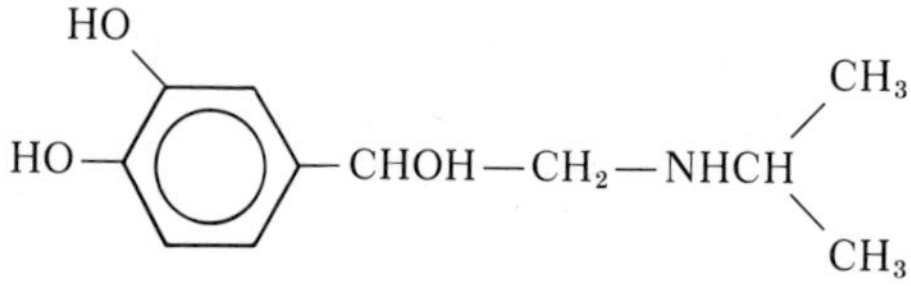

Isoproterenol

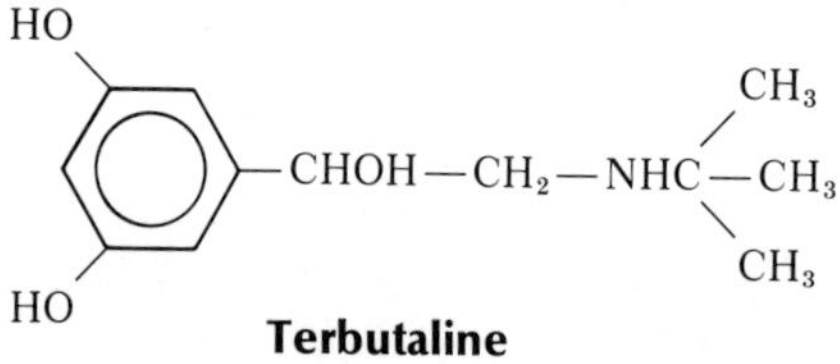

Terbutaline

Fig. 1. Adding more hydrocarbon groups to the terminal amino portion of the molecule confers beta adrenergic specificity. Epinephrine is both alpha and beta adrenergic, isoproterenol is almost purely beta adrenergic, whereas terbutaline is predominantly beta$_2$ adrenergic.

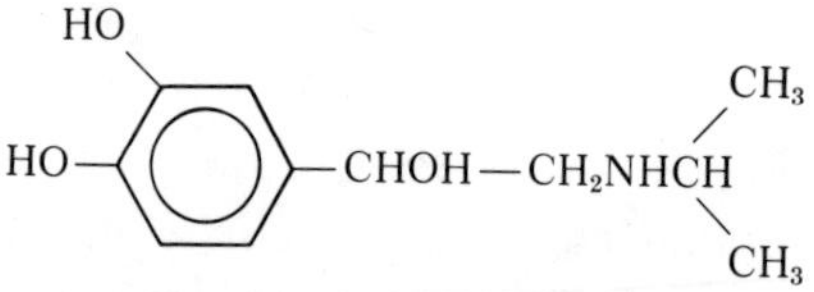

Isoproterenol (beta adrenergic)

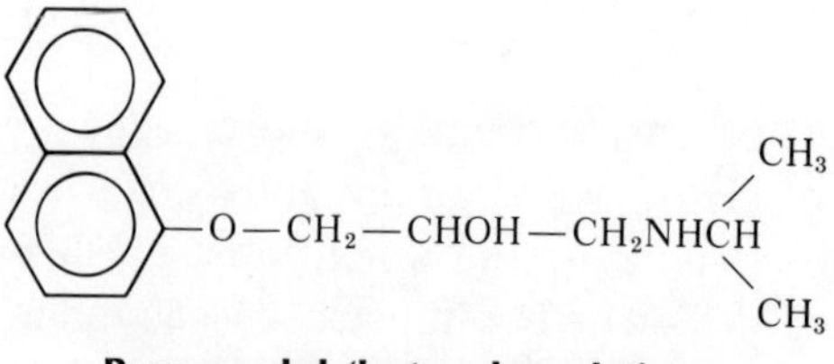

Propranolol (beta adrenolytic)

Fig. 2. The structural similarity of beta adrenergic (agonist) and beta adrenolytic (antagonist) drugs is exemplified by isoproterenol and propranolol.

vent or diminish the activity of an agonist; such a drug is an *antagonist*. Often the molecular conformation of an antagonist closely resembles the conformation of the corresponding agonist, as shown in Fig. 2. *Specificity.* A few generalizations can be drawn from the drug-receptor concept. Where there is but a single bond or bonding is weak, specificity is limited and the allowable variations in chemical structure are large. This is exemplified by the sedative-hypnotic class of drugs, to which bromides, alcohols, and barbiturates belong. Not only are these chemically quite different, but considerable alteration of molecular structure in each category is permissible without marked loss of efficacy. Also considerable variation in the side actions of each group is observed.

Multiple-bonding drugs, on the other hand, are likely to show more clearly definable structural characteristics. If there are three or more bonds, the three-dimensional nature of the molecule is critical and stereoisomers may show marked differences in activity. Epinephrine is a familiar example; its *l*-isomer has about a hundred times the bronchodilator potency of its *d*-isomer (Fig. 3). The drug class is much more clearly circumscribed, and side actions may be so similar that a definite pharmacologic "syndrome" can be described. The remarkable similarity of action of morphinoids and related narcotics is a reflection of the high specificity of multiple bonding. Both

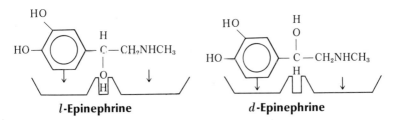

l-Epinephrine   *d*-Epinephrine

Fig. 3. The *l*-epinephrine molecule fits the hypothetical receptor site more accurately than does the *d*-epinephrine molecule. The bronchodilator potency of the *l*-isomer is about a hundred times that of the *d*-isomer.

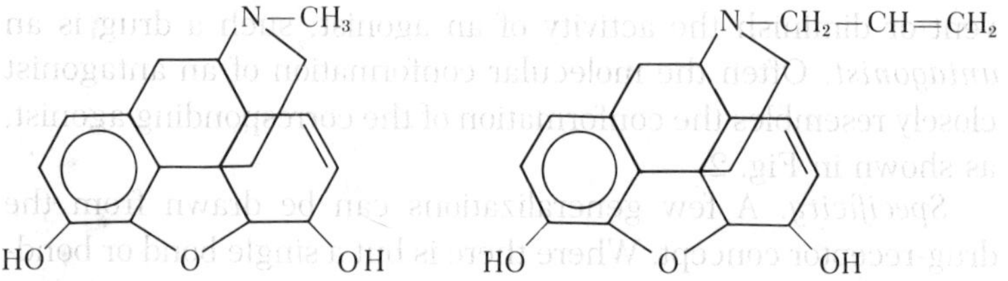

Morphine (agonist)   **Nalorphine (antagonist)**

Fig. 4. The close chemical similarity between agonist and antagonist reflects the high specificity of narcotic molecules.

agonists (narcotics) and antagonists (antinarcotics) possess molecular configurations that are readily identifiable (Fig. 4).

Toxicity

Each drug approved for clinical use has a standard *dose,* which is the amount required to produce the desired therapeutic effect in the average-sized adult. When this dose is exceeded, toxic properties usually appear. Large overdoses may be fatal. A convenient measure of the toxicity of a drug is the ratio of the lethal dose to the therapeutic dose; this is called the *therapeutic index.* Dosage tolerances may vary widely among individuals. Unusual sensitivity to the action of a drug is sometimes termed *idiosyncrasy.* A chemical impurity may contribute to toxic activity. All drugs approved by the Food and Drug Administration include in their descriptions the required standards of purity.

Toxic side actions may be inherent in the drug itself or may result from formation of toxic metabolic products. Methyl alcohol is relatively innocuous; but when it is oxidized in the liver, formaldehyde and formic acid are produced and these are highly poisonous. Frequently toxic actions may be directed to certain organs, particularly the liver, kidney, bone marrow, and central nervous system.

Another disturbance commonly observed after prolonged use of antibiotics is *superinfection,* the overgrowth of bacterial or fungal species that are unaffected by the drug.

Allergy

Drugs may act as *antigens* (i.e., may stimulate the formation of specific immunoglobulins, called *antibodies*). Subsequent administrations of the drug are then followed by an antigen-antibody reaction with tissue destruction and the release of physiologically active products, including histamine and serotonin, both of which are powerful bronchoconstrictors. This is the phenomenon of drug allergy, involving not only the respiratory tract (laryngospasm, wheezing) but all other organ systems as well. Skin manifestations (e.g., hives, eczema) are well known. The gastrointestinal tract, kidney, liver, or bone marrow may be similarly involved. In severe reactions there may be widespread capillary dilatation, loss of circulating volume, and shock. This is termed *anaphylaxis*.

Resistance

Frequently a patient is encountered whose response to a drug is diminished or absent. Drug resistance may be inherited or acquired by habituation, or by cross-tolerance through prolonged use of a closely similar drug. Asthmatic patients may become tolerant to bronchodilators, and the drugs may no longer be effective when needed. Tolerance may be acquired very rapidly, total resistance being attained after only a few doses. This is occasionally seen with epinephrine employed as an emergency bronchodilator. The phenomenon is termed *tachyphylaxis*.

Synergism and antagonism

When more than one drug is administered to achieve a therapeutic effect, the combination may be additive (i.e., the sum of the individual actions); or a greater activity may occur than the sum of the actions of the drugs would indicate. This is usually termed drug *synergism,* and the action of one is said to be potentiated by the action of the other. A well-known example is the synergism shown by epinephrine and aminophylline when these agents are used together in the treatment of asthma.

Drugs may also be *antagonistic*, the effect of one tending to cancel that of the other. Antagonism may result simply from the fact that the dominant actions of the drugs are opposed, as might be seen after the combined administration of a sedative and a stimulant. Instances are known, however, in which the drug antagonist actually displaces or substitutes itself for the drug. An example is nalorphine, a drug closely related to morphine; nalorphine will inhibit the action of morphine presumably by replacing morphine molecules at their sites of action. This type of antagonism is often termed *competitive inhibition.*

Factors determining duration of effect

Drug action may be terminated by elimination of the drug from the body either unchanged or in metabolized form; or there may be redistribution and the drug may be sequestered in fat or other tissue where it exerts no effect. Tachyphylaxis or administration of an antagonist will also terminate drug action.

Many patient factors are important in determining the anticipated effect of a drug. Besides age, sex, nutrition, and pathologic conditions—there are psychologic factors, depending on the temperament and attitude of the patient during therapy. Suggestion may play a significant role in determining the desirable response to medication. This *placebo* effect may be difficult to evaluate and may result in the continued use of a worthless or inactive preparation.

Motor systems

Many drugs exert their effects on somatic and autonomic motor systems. Somatic innervation supplies skeletal muscle; autonomic nerves supply cardiac and smooth muscle and the secretory activity of exocrine glands. Smooth muscle is present throughout the organ systems of the body—especially in bronchi, blood vessels, and the gastrointestinal, biliary, and genitourinary tracts. Of particular importance in respiratory therapy are drugs that alter smooth muscle tone in the bronchioles or drugs that affect the muscles of respiration. A brief discussion of the transmission of nerve impulses in motor systems may be helpful.

Physiology of the somatic system. Motor fibers that supply skeletal muscle arise in the anterior horn cells of the spinal gray matter. Origins of motor fibers of the cranial nerves are found in the midbrain and medulla. A single nerve fiber conducts the impulse from the central nervous system to the muscle site. At the junction of nerve and muscle, a complex electrochemical process occurs involving the release of a transmitter substance, acetylcholine. The presence or absence of this chemical mediator is of great physiologic importance, and facilitation of or interference with its action is the principal pharmacologic approach to skeletal muscle paralysis or restoration of muscle tone.

Physiology of the autonomic system. The autonomic system is separable into two divisions, parasympathetic and sympathetic.

The *parasympathetic* system is concerned chiefly with metabolic and excretory functions (i.e., with the normal processes of the body economy). Anatomically, parasympathetic nerve fibers arise in the midbrain or brain stem or from the sacral cord. The name *craniosacral* is occasionally applied to the parasympathetic system.

Transmission from the central nervous system requires a two-neuron relay. The first neuron proceeds from the central nervous system to a ganglion, a neuronal structure usually lying quite close to the organ innervated. The second neuron proceeds from the ganglion to the smooth muscle, cardiac muscle, or exocrine gland structure. Transmission both at the synapse between the first and second neurons in the ganglion and at the neuroeffector junction is mediated by acetylcholine.

The *sympathetic* system has been described as the alarm system of the organism, mobilizing the organism's metabolic resources to cope with environmental threats. Smooth muscle and glandular activities cease, cardiac activity is stimulated, and blood supply to skeletal muscle is augmented. In contrast to the parasympathetic system, which tends to act by discrete and individual parts in response to specific needs of the organism, the sympathetic system tends to discharge as a unit, producing a mass effect. Cannon[1] summarized this distinction by the following analogy: "The sympathetics are like the loud and soft pedals of a piano, modulating all the notes together; the parasympathetic innervations are like the separate keys."

Sympathetic innervation also involves a two-neuron relay,

with the first neurons arising from the gray matter of the thoracic and lumbar cord. Hence the term *thoracolumbar* is occasionally used to designate this autonomic division. The first neurons synapse with the second neurons in the ganglia, and the impulse is propagated to the neuroeffector junction. Ganglionic transmission is mediated by acetylcholine; and some neuroeffector junctions utilize acetylcholine as a mediator (chiefly the sweat glands). At the majority of neuroeffector sites, however, the chemical transmitter is another substance belonging to a group of compounds known as catecholamines; these include dopamine, norepinephrine, and epinephrine.

Autonomic drugs

The discovery of neurohumoral transmission provided a unifying theory on which the classification of autonomic and muscle relaxant drugs could be conveniently organized.

As just noted, acetylcholine mediates nerve impulses both in the autonomic ganglia and at the myoneural junctions. These connections are similar morphologically and physiologically. Acetylcholine is liberated, mediates the nerve impulse, and is destroyed with "flashlike suddenness" (Dale[2]) by a specific enzyme—acetylcholinesterase. Transmission at these sites is distinguished by extreme rapidity, the duration of action being on the order of 0.001 second. Since the phenomena are elicited by small doses of nicotine, they are referred to as the *nicotinic* actions of acetylcholine.

Transmission is also mediated by acetylcholine at all parasympathetic neuroeffector junctions and at sympathetic endings in the sweat glands. Conduction is slower at these sites, and the action of acetylcholine is more prolonged. The effects are produced by muscarine, a substance closely similar to acetylcholine found in poisonous mushrooms, and are termed *muscarinic* actions.

Drugs that mimic the action of acetylcholine are termed *cholinergic*. They may elicit their phenomena according to either or both of the two principal patterns, nicotinic and muscarinic.

Drugs that antagonize the action of acetylcholine are termed *anticholinergic*. Those which interfere with transmission in the autonomic ganglia are called *gangliolytic;* those which oppose conduction at the myoneural junction of skeletal muscle are usually referred to as paralyzants or *myoneural blocking agents.* Gangliolytic drugs are used for control of blood pressure; an example is trimethaphan (Arfonad). Myoneural blocking agents are more fully described in Chapter 4.

Drugs that mimic sympathetic activity are termed *adrenergic* and are divided into two distinct groups. Those which resemble norepinephrine are *alpha adrenergic.* They are distinguished chiefly by vasoconstrictor activity and comprise the drugs employed as bronchial mucosal decongestants, such as phenylephrine. The other type, designated *beta adrenergic,* more closely resemble epinephrine, the hormonal product of the adrenal medulla. Their activities are principally smooth muscle relaxant and cardiac muscle stimulant. A typical beta adrenergic drug is isoproterenol, which relaxes bronchial smooth muscle and increases the rate and force of cardiac contraction (Table 2-1).

A further division has been made more recently between beta receptors to cardiac muscle *(beta₁)* and those affecting smooth muscle structures *(beta₂).* From this observation, research efforts are being directed toward the development of bronchodilator drugs with diminished cardiac effects (i.e., compounds that have pronounced beta₂ action but that produce minimal beta₁ responses).

The duration of action of catecholamines is generally short; a single dose is effective for 2 to 3 minutes as a rule. The catechol

nucleus (HO—⟨◯⟩—) is rapidly methylated (HO—⟨◯⟩—),
         HO   CH₃O

a reaction catalyzed by the enzyme catechol *ortho*-methyl transferase (COMT). The methylation of catechol accounts for the evanescent action of isoproterenol and isoetharine. When the catechol configuration is lacking (as in metaproterenol, terbutaline, and ephedrine), the in vivo stability is increased and the bronchodilator activity prolonged.

Drugs that interfere with sympathetic neuroeffector trans-

Table 1-2. Drugs affecting motor systems*

Cholinergic		Adrenergic		
Nicotinic	Muscarine	Alpha	Beta$_1$	Beta$_2$

Acetylcholine
Methacholine
Anticholinesterases
  Neostigmine
  Pyridostigmine
  Edrophonium
		←————————Epinephrine————————→
		Norepinephrine
		←————————Ephedrine————————→
		Phenylephrine
		Cyclopentamine
		  ←————Isoproterenol——→
		  ←————Isoetharine——→
		  ←————Terbutaline→		

Anticholinergic			Adrenolytic	
Gangliolytic	Myoneural blocking	Anti-muscarinic	Alpha	Beta
Trimethaphan	d-Tubocurarine Gallamine Pancuronium Succinylcholine	Atropine Sch 1,000 (ipratro- pium)	Phenotolamine	Propranolol

*See also Table 2-1.

mission are termed *adrenolytic*. Both alpha and beta adrenolytic compounds are known; indeed, there is little overlap between the actions of these two groups of drugs. An example of a beta adrenolytic drug is propranolol, used in the treatment of cardiac arrhythmias. Due to blockade of the beta adrenergic activity in the bronchi, propranolol may produce serious bronchospasm in patients with asthma. The alpha adrenolytic drug phentolamine has been used as a bronchodilator, although its action may be unrelated to its sympathetic activity.

Some autonomic and neuromuscular drugs discussed are classified in Table 1-2.

REFERENCES

1. Cannon, W. B.: The wisdom of the body, New York, 1932, W. W. Norton & Co., Inc.
2. Dale, H. H.: Transmission of nervous effects by acetylcholine, Harvey Lect. **32:**229-245, 1937.
3. Goldstein, A., Aronow, L., and Kalman, S. M.: Principles of drug action; the basis of pharmacology, ed. 2, New York, 1974, John Wiley & Sons, Inc.

4. Goodman, L. S., and Gilman, A., editors: The pharmacological basis of therapeutics, ed. 5, New York, 1975, Macmillan Publishing Co., Inc.
5. Levine, R. R.: Pharmacology; drug actions and reactions, Boston, 1973, Little, Brown & Co.
6. Melmon, K. L., and Morrelli, H. F., editors: Clinical pharmacology; basic principles in therapeutics, New York, 1972, Macmillan Publishing Co., Inc.

OFFICIAL DRUG COMPENDIA

American drug index, 1976. (Wilson, C. O., and Jones, T. E., editors.) Philadelphia, 1976, J. B. Lippincott Co.

The national formulary, XIV (American Pharmaceutical Association), Easton, Pa., 1974, Mack Printing Co. (Became official 1975.)

The pharmacopeia of the United States of America, XIX revised (The United States Pharmacopeial Convention, Inc.), Easton, Pa., 1974, Mack Printing Co. (Became official 1975.)

2 Bronchoactive drugs

Mechanisms of bronchoconstriction

Bronchial mucosal irritation (due to particulate matter, chemical irritants, or thermal changes) induces smooth muscle spasm, preventing access of harmful substances to the lower airways. Reflex responses of this type are appropriate if bronchial lumina are not overconstricted; however, marked increases in airway resistance will greatly increase the work of breathing.

Bronchoconstriction produced by allergens or by inflammatory responses to pathogens is compounded by edema formation. Products of tissue reaction (e.g., histamine, serotonin, plasma kinins) provoke hyperemia and swelling of the bronchial mucosa. Inflammatory exudates and hypersecretion of mucus tend to fill the airways and further interfere with gas exchange. Certain drugs may evoke bronchoconstrictor responses as undesirable side effects. Cholinergic agents (e.g., neostigmine) employed to reverse the effects of muscle relaxants in anesthesia, comprise one such class. Propranolol, a beta adrenergic blocking agent used to combat ventricular arrhythmias, may also provoke bronchospasm.

The problem is thus a composite of several factors. Bronchodilatation may require relaxation of bronchial smooth muscle, bronchial mucosal decongestion, and inhibition of secretory activity. Suppression of secretions may predispose to formation of mucus plugs but will be effective if the patient is well hydrated.

Role of cyclic 3'-5' AMP in beta adrenergic activity.[4] Intracellular biochemical changes accompanying beta activity involve the conversion of an energy-rich compound, adenosine triphosphate (ATP), to adenosine monophosphate (AMP). This biodegradation provides much of the free energy essential to effector function. An intermediary substance of great importance in this system is cyclic 3'-5' AMP, which is so closely linked to beta activity that it has in the past been described as the receptor itself. Although the concept is oversimplified, the appearance of cyclic AMP accompanies beta stimulation. Probably cyclic AMP is an essential chemical messenger operating within the effector cell.

Cyclic AMP formation is catalyzed by an enzyme system located in the effector cell membrane. The principal enzyme, adenylate cyclase, can be induced (i.e., its formation can be stimulated) by epinephrine and other catecholamines. The resulting increase in cyclic AMP formation initiates the intracellular reactions essential to relaxation of bronchial smooth muscle.

Aided by another enzyme, phosphodiesterase, cyclic 3'-5' AMP is converted to 5'-AMP. The phosphodiesterase is inhibited by a class of compounds known as methylxanthines, which include aminophylline. Both adenylate cyclase induction and phosphodiesterase inhibition tend to favor cyclic AMP buildup; and this buildup may account for the bronchodilator activity of catecholamines and methylxanthines.

The reactions can be simply represented as follows:

$$ATP \xrightarrow[\text{[Mg}^{++}\text{]}]{\text{Adenylate cyclase}} \text{Cyclic 3'-5' AMP} \xrightarrow[\text{[Mg}^{++}\text{]}]{\text{Phosphodiesterase}} 5' AMP$$

(induced by   (inhibited by
catecholamines)   methylxanthines)

The intracellular level of cyclic AMP may be depressed by alpha adrenergic stimulation, cholinergic stimulation (e.g., with methacholine), or beta adrenergic blockade (with propranolol).[21,31]

Mediator release. The asthma attack is characterized by the release of several substances, termed *mediators,* which are disparate chemically but any one of which can trigger an episode of bronchospasm. They include histamine, serotonin, and acetylcholine (all chemical transmitters in the nervous system) and slow-reactive substance of anaphylaxis (SRS-A) (a peptide of much greater complexity).[20,25] Part of the difficulty in asthma management is related to the fact that a single drug is likely to antagonize or inhibit the action of only one mediator. Antihistamines and antiserotonins generally have little effect.

According to Townley,[33] a common feature observed in asthmatic patients is marked sensitivity to nebulized methacholine, a closely related congener of acetylcholine. Remember: acetylcholine is the chemical transmitter at the ends of parasympathetic nerves to bronchial smooth muscle cells that causes the muscle to constrict when stimulated. Normally this action is opposed by release of catecholamines from the sympathetic innervation.

Relatively large doses of methacholine are required to produce bronchoconstriction in the normal individual. The asthmatic patient, however, develops bronchospasm after inhalation of one hundredth or one thousandth this amount. Animal and human studies have shown that the phenomenon occurs after beta adrenergic blockade, suggesting that asthmatic patients may be in a state of autonomic imbalance with parasympathetic dominance largely unopposed. When beta adrenergic receptors are blocked, sensitivity to many bronchoconstrictor substances is demonstrable—including histamine, serotonin, and prostaglandin F_2 alpha. Thus partial beta blockade may be the underlying deficiency that causes the asthmatic patient to react strongly to endogenously produced bronchoactive metabolites.

Adrenergic drugs (Table 2-1)

Depending on the nature of the autonomic effector cell, sympathetic stimulation produces two distinct bronchiolar effects. The so-called alpha receptors evoke a response that is vasoconstrictor; beta receptors cause relaxation of bronchial smooth muscle. Adrenergic drugs may elicit either alpha or beta responses, or both.

Drugs acting primarily on alpha receptors. The use of vasoconstrictor substances in the tracheobronchial tree is analogous to their use as nasal decongestants. Thus phenylephrine (Neo-Synephrine) is employed in nose drops and may be given by aerosol to promote shrinkage of the bronchial mucosa. Cyclopentamine (Clopane) is a congener of propylhexedrine (Benzedrex), the well-known nasal decongestant. Cyclopentamine is combined with isoproterenol in the aerosol preparation Aerolone Compound. A number of similar combinations of alpha adrenergic and beta adrenergic drugs are available for administration by nebulizer. Bronkosol contains phenylephrine and the $beta_2$ active compound isoetharine.

Preparations of bronchodilators, with their dose ranges for aerosol administration, are shown in Table 2-2.

Drugs acting primarily on beta receptors. These are the bronchodilators most familiar to the therapist. For treatment of asthma attacks, to promote mobilization of retained secretions, and to facilitate the evaluation of pulmonary function, beta adrenergic compounds are usually selected. Their effectiveness when administered by aerosol places added responsibility on the therapist for their safe employment.

The sympathetic receptors of the heart belong mostly to the beta category. Thus beta adrenergic drugs are likely to produce an increase in the rate and force of myocardial contraction. Such activity may be therapeutically useful, but it also may be dangerous in the presence of heart disease. Perhaps the chief hazard associated with the use of beta adrenergic compounds is increased irritability of the cardiac conduction network, causing tachyarrhythmias or ventricular fibrillation.

Studies have demonstrated a difference between beta receptors in the heart and beta receptors in smooth muscle structures.[18] The two types are designated $beta_1$ and $beta_2$, respectively. Selective response of either type is thus theoretically possible, and a bronchodilator ($beta_2$) effect can be obtained with less cardiotonic ($beta_1$) side effects. Salbutamol and terbutaline possess marked $beta_2$ but much weaker $beta_1$ activities.

Epinephrine (adrenaline) is a product of the adrenal medulla that occurs naturally as the *l*-isomer. It shows pronounced alpha and beta effects, the latter being more prolonged. The decongestant (vasopressor) effect may actually be reversed as the alpha response diminishes and the vasodilator beta action remains. Secretory activity is inhibited, but a sympathomimetic action produces viscid saliva.

Toxic effects include tachycardia, palpitation, hypertension,

Table 2-1. Catecholamines and related adrenergic drugs

Catecholamines				
Epinephrine		OH	CH_3	
Norepinephrine		OH	H	
Dopamine		H	H	
Alpha adrenergic decongestants				
Phenylephrine	3—OH	OH	H	CH_3
Cyclopentamine		H	CH_3	CH_3
Propylhexedrine		H	CH_3	CH_3
Beta adrenergic bronchodilators				
Ephedrine		OH	CH_3	CH_3

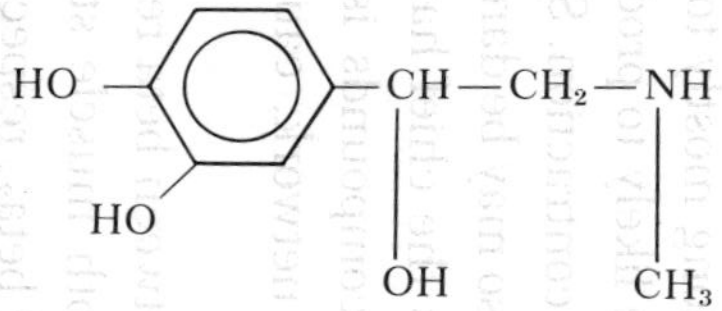

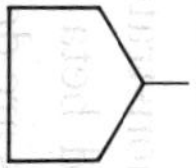

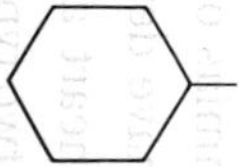

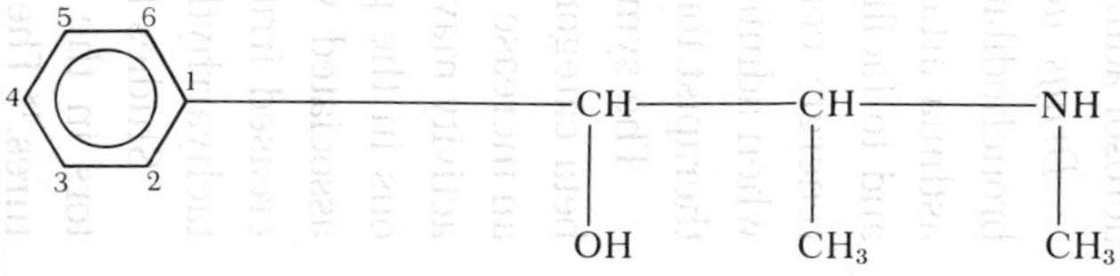

Drug				
Isoproterenol	3—OH, 4—OH	OH	H	CH(CH$_3$)$_2$
Isoetharine	3—OH, 4—OH	OH	CH$_2$CH$_3$	CH(CH$_3$)$_2$
Metaproterenol	3—OH, 5—OH	OH	H	CH(CH$_3$)$_2$
Terbutaline	3—OH, 5—OH	OH	H	C(CH$_3$)$_3$
Fenoterol	3—OH, 5—OH	OH	H	CH(CH$_3$)—CH$_2$—C$_6$H$_4$(4—OH)
Ritodrine	4—OH	OH	CH$_3$	CH$_2$CH$_2$—C$_6$H$_4$(4—OH)
Methoxyphenamine	2—OCH$_3$	H	CH$_3$	CH$_3$
Salbutamol	3—CH$_2$OH, 4—OH	OH	H	C(CH$_3$)$_3$
Soterenol	3—NHSO$_2$CH$_3$, 4—OH	OH	H	CH(CH$_3$)$_2$
Quinterenol	(8-hydroxyquinolin-5-yl)	OH	H	CH(CH$_3$)$_2$

Table 2-2. Recommended doses of aerosolized bronchodilators

	Hand nebulizer (number of inhalations)	Compressor, IPPB (ml)
Racemic epinephrine (1.25%)	2-3	0.3-1
Isoproterenol (0.5%)	5-15	0.5
Isoproterenol (0.25%) with cyclopentamine (0.5%) (Aerolone Compound)	6-12	(not recommended)
Isoetharine (1.0%) with phenylephrine (0.25%) (Bronkosol)	3-7	0.25-1

headache, sweating, anxiety, and tremor. Epinephrine must be used with great caution in patients with cardiovascular disease.

Synthetic epinephrine is a mixture of equal parts of *l*- and *d*-isomers (racemic epinephrine); *d*-epinephrine has about 1% the beta adrenergic effect of the *l*-derivative. Racemic epinephrine thus has about half the action of an equal dose of the pure *l*-isomer.

Isoproterenol is produced by substitution of an N-isopropyl group for the N-methyl group of epinephrine. It is a powerful beta adrenergic compound with little or no alpha activity. Like other catecholamines, it is ultra–short acting. Since it is prepared synthetically, it is a racemic mixture; however, its *l*-isomer has 300 to 600 times the beta activity of its *d*-isomer. It is one of the most potent cardiotonic substances known and is hazardous to use in the patient with preexisting heart disease. Side effects are similar to those observed with epinephrine.

Preparations are available which combine isoproterenol with an alpha adrenergic drug, such as phenylephrine (Duo-Medihaler) or cyclopentamine (Aerolone Compound). The topical vasoconstriction reduces systemic absorption and consequent side actions.[13]

Isoetharine (Dilabron)[5,8] is the ethyl homologue of isoproterenol; the substitution reduces beta$_1$ adrenergic activity to about a sixteenth. Alpha effects are wanting. The action of isoetharine on bronchial smooth muscle is comparable to that of epinephrine. The drug is marketed in combination with phenylephrine (Bronkosol-2).

Beta$_2$ adrenergic compounds. Selective stimulant action on beta$_2$ receptors permits the relaxation of smooth muscle structures with less risk of cardiotonic side effects. Several such compounds have been developed; alphabetically, they include the following:

1. Fenoterol (Berotec)
2. Isoetharine (Dilabron)[5,8]
3. Metaproterenol (Alupent, Orciprenaline)[5]
4. Quinterenol (Quinprenaline)
5. Ritodrine (Premar)
6. Salbutamol (Albuterol, Ventolin)[1,19]
7. Soterenol
8. Terbutaline (Brethine, Bricanyl)[2,27]

Isoetharine is the only catecholamine; thus it is susceptible to COMT, which shortens its duration of action. The others are relatively long acting; their bronchodilator effects generally persist for about 4 hours. Metaproterenol is an isomer of isoproterenol but with the phenolic hydroxyl groups in the 3,5 positions (a resorcinol). The drug therefore is resistant to COMT but possesses substantial beta activity. Terbutaline, another resorcinol, is the *tert*-butyl homologue of metaproterenol; it is somewhat stabler and longer acting.

Metaproterenol, salbutamol, and terbutaline can be administered orally. Metaproterenol is available as 20 mg tablets, terbutaline as 5 mg tablets. The recommended dose schedule is one tablet 3 or 4 times/day. Nervousness, tremor, and weakness are common side actions; occasionally drowsiness is observed.

Ephedrine is a much more stable but less potent adrenergic compound with predominantly beta activity. It can be given by injection, but its greatest usefulness as a bronchodilator lies in its efficacy by the oral route. Dosage ranges from 15 to 50 mg. Since it possesses central stimulant properties, ephedrine is combined with sedatives (e.g., barbiturates) in a number of drug preparations for control of asthma in the ambulatory patient. A space isomer of ephedrine, termed *pseudoephedrine* (Sudafed), is marketed for use as an oral decongestant.

Methoxyphenamine and *metaproterenol* are available in oral preparations; they are effective bronchodilators without significant stimulant activity.

Clinical use of bronchodilators administered by aerosol[22,29]

The immediate need for bronchodilation is the principal indication for administration by aerosol. Adrenergic drugs are almost exclusively employed. Absorption from mucous surfaces is rapid, approaching the serial blood values that would be obtained after intravenous administration. Although relatively small doses are required, only 5% to 10% of the aerosolized drug reaches the site of action. Some is absorbed from the pharynx and may contribute to systemic toxicity. Doubtless the occurrence of undesirable effects after aerosol administration is due in large part to drug which is swallowed. Rinsing the mouth is a useful routine after the aerosol treatment. Dosage ranges are wide, particularly with the catecholamine derivatives, whose duration of action is short. Tachycardia and tachyarrhythmia must be avoided by constant attention to pulse rate and volume. ECG monitoring is essential in the patient with an irritable heart. Every effort must be made, through measurements of forced expired volume in 1 second ($FEV_{1.0}$) or of peak flow, to demonstrate the efficacy of treatment.

Many factors—mechanical, physiologic, and psychologic— determine the efficacy of bronchodilator therapy. Patient cooperation is essential. Penetration of nebulized particles can occur only if airways are reasonably patent and inspiratory flows sufficient to draw particles into the finer bronchioles.

Fig. 5 summarizes some of the factors determining the therapeutic response of the patient.

Pressurized aerosols. Preparations containing epinephrine or isoproterenol are marketed in pressurized containers employing a chlorofluorinated hydrocarbon (Freon) as the propellant. Indiscriminate use of these aerosols may have resulted in an increased mortality from asthma in the 1960s. Some deaths were due to tachyarrhythmias or ventricular fibrillation. In some instances, the propellant may sensitize the myocardium to the arrhythmogenic action of catecholamines.[7,14,28,32]

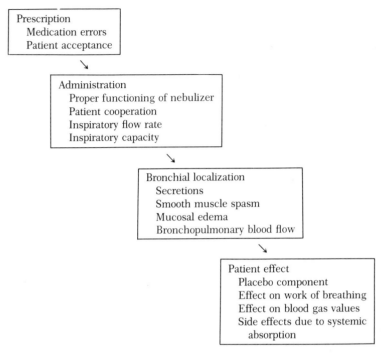

Fig. 5. Factors influencing effects of bronchodilators given by aerosol.

Alpha adrenolytic drugs. As the name would suggest, these are compounds with vasodilator activity that are employed clinically for the treatment of peripheral vascular disease. Some of them have significant bronchodilator properties. Phentolamine (Regitine) has been administered in aerosolized form for treatment of asthma.[12]

Anticholinergic drugs. Compounds that block transmission at parasympathetic neuroeffector junctions promote smooth muscle relaxation and inhibition of secretory activity. Atropine, an alkaloid found in belladonna leaves, has been used by aerosol for relief of asthma. Inhibition of secretions, with drying and mucus plug formation, may occur but can be minimized by adequate hydration of the patient. A new derivative of atropine, Sch 1,000 (ipratropium), has fewer side effects per dose. It is now being tested as an aerosol for clinical use.[30]

Methylxanthines. These include the familiar compounds

present in stimulant beverages—caffeine (coffee, tea, cola), theobromine (cocoa), and theophylline (tea). All are methylated derivatives of the natural metabolite xanthine, a precursor of uric acid. Aside from their central stimulating effects, methylxanthines possess a number of properties that are clinically useful. They are employed as diuretics and as coronary vasodilators. All have bronchodilator activity, but only theophylline is employed therapeutically for this purpose.

Aminophylline (theophylline ethylenediamine)[24] is a conjugate of 78% anhydrous theophylline and 12% ethylenediamine. The latter is added to render theophylline water soluble. It may be given orally, rectally, or by injection in doses of 0.25 to 0.5 gm. Its action is relatively slow but well adapted for continuous use since side actions are relatively benign. It can be given slowly intravenously; an infusion consisting of 0.5 gm/500 ml of solution is convenient. The drug is a vasodilator, and marked hypotension may be produced if administration is rapid. Other side effects that may appear include nausea, vomiting, tremor, nervousness, and tachycardia.

Corticosteroids. Perhaps no class of drugs presently in use has the wide spectrum of activity exhibited by corticotropin (ACTH) and the steroids elaborated by the adrenal cortex. Their suppressant effects on immunologic diseases such as asthma are well known but poorly understood. They interfere with the release of histamine, however, and effectively antagonize the inflammatory process.[3,34] They enhance resistance to stress and fortify the surgical patient against the deleterious influences of trauma, shock, and anesthesia. These beneficial effects are counterbalanced by the protein catabolism they produce, which causes reduction of tissue resistance and may lead to gastrointestinal ulceration or spread of existing infection.

Thus, when defensive tissue response is suppressed, susceptibility to pathogenic invaders is increased. The patient who has received corticosteroids over an extended period will suffer from adrenal insufficiency unless medication is continued, since atrophy of the adrenal cortex occurs. This individual is particularly susceptible to stress and may go into acute circulatory collapse if he is injured or becomes ill. Declining blood pressure, weakness and faintness, and nausea and vomiting are the symptoms and signs of adrenal failure (addisonian crisis); and these will not be relieved until corticosteroids are administered.

Prolonged corticosteroid excess results in a syndrome known as hypercorticism, or Cushing's syndrome—characterized by obesity, hyperglycemia, wasting of muscles, acne, and masculinizing signs in women.

Corticosteroids (e.g., hydrocortisone, dexamethasone, prednisolone, methylprednisolone, triamcinolone) are helpful in terminating an acute asthma attack and in relieving the disabling symptoms of chronic bronchial asthma.[11] Their side effects, principally alterations in the metabolism of proteins and carbohydrates and in the distribution of electrolytes, are serious enough to preclude their use when other measures can be employed. A single intravenous injection of a corticosteroid is probably not harmful, however, and may be less provocative of toxic manifestations than an injection of epinephrine or isoproterenol. Onset of action is slow, requiring at least 30 minutes for maximum effect. Therefore these compounds are less useful in emergency situations than are beta adrenergic drugs.

Aerosolized corticosteroids have been advocated for treatment of asthma attacks. Hydrocortisone is largely ineffective, but dexamethasone and triamcinolone can be given satisfactorily by inhalation. Significant systemic absorption occurs, however, and it may be contended that the parenteral route is easier to employ and produces bronchodilatation just as rapidly. A newer derivative, beclomethasone dipropionate, is a corticosteroid with a powerful topical action. The drug may be effective in a daily dose of 0.4 mg without biochemical evidence of significant adrenal suppression[10]; but subsequent use has revealed instances of adrenal insufficiency.[16] Beclomethasone dipropionate (Vanceril) is available for use by inhaler. The adult dosage recommended is two inhalations 3 to 4 times/day, with maximal daily intake not to exceed 1 mg.

Antihistamines. Chronic bronchial asthma usually exhibits the characteristics of an allergic response, manifested by the bronchoconstriction and bronchial edema produced by histamine; but antihistamines are effective only in mild asthma

episodes. Even then, tolerance to the drugs is rapidly acquired
and effectiveness is lost. Also the drugs possess anticholinergic
activity, promoting the suppression of secretions and mucus plug
formation. Hydroxyzine (Atarax, Vistaril) is an antihistamine
often prescribed as a sedative or for relief of anxiety; it has some
bronchodilator effect.[15]

Nitrites. Any drug that depresses smooth muscle may have
bronchodilator efficacy. Nitrites are generally employed as coronary and systemic vasodilators, but they have been tried for
nearly all types of smooth muscle spasm. Nitroglycerin, employed
sublingually as for angina pectoris, may provide relief in an acute
asthma attack.

Cromolyn.[9,17,23] This compound (Aarane, Intal) represents a
new development in the management of chronic bronchial
asthma. It apparently inhibits the degranulation of sensitized
pulmonary mast cells, thus preventing the release of histamine
and SRS-A on exposure to antigen.[26] It has no bronchodilator,
antihistaminic, or anti-inflammatory action of its own. It is ineffective when given during acute asthma and must be viewed
solely as a preventive drug. Administration is by inhalation of the
powdered compound directly into the airways. Capsules containing 20 mg of cromolyn are available; the recommended dose
schedule is 4 times/day. A special inhaler is provided that
punctures the capsule and disperses the powder with a small
propellor on inhalation. Beneficial effects may not be observed
until treatments have been given for 2 to 4 weeks.

Acute asthma

In susceptible individuals, wheezing with progressive dyspnea may accompany exposure to lung irritants, temperature
changes, or dusts. Attacks may be precipitated by upper respiratory infection. Of particular interest are the allergic responses
that may follow administration of drugs. Antibiotics of the
penicillin group are notorious; all patients who receive these or
similar medications must be questioned specifically concerning
previous untoward reactions. Aspirin sensitivity is present in a
significant percentage of patients with chronic asthma.

The asthma attack is often initiated by a paroxysm of coughing followed by bronchospasm, mucosal edema, and the production of viscid secretions. Work of breathing is markedly increased, and dyspnea may be severe. Air becomes trapped in the alveoli; overdistention occurs, and the chest is fixed in the inspiratory position. Expiration is difficult and prolonged. The accessory muscles of respiration (trapezius, sternocleidomastoid) are employed. The tenacious mucoid sputum intensifies the discomfort, and further bouts of coughing contribute to additional bronchospasm and mucosal congestion.

Treatment of asthma. Acute episodes of asthma are usually relieved within 5 minutes after a few breaths of nebulized racemic epinephrine (1%), isoproterenol (0.5% to 1%), metaproterenol (5%), or isoetharine (1%) with phenylephrine (0.25%) (Bronkosol). Maximal expiratory flow and vital capacity are improved; however, ventilation-perfusion imbalance may not be corrected and the Pa_{O_2} may remain unchanged or even decrease. Treatments may need to be repeated at 5-minute intervals until relief is obtained.

Alternatively 0.2 to 0.5 mg of epinephrine can be injected subcutaneously, and its absorption hastened by massage. This can be repeated at 15- to 20-minute intervals without cumulative effect, but tolerance is rapidly acquired and the dose may need to be increased. Administration of intravenous infusions containing epinephrine is hazardous and is no longer recommended. Aminophylline (0.5 gm) may be given in 10 to 20 ml of normal saline slowly intravenously or in a 500 ml infusion by drip.

A severe attack requires not only immediate bronchodilator therapy but also oxygen and occasionally continuous mechanical ventilation. Adequate hydration with intravenous fluids is essential for mobilization of secretions. Intermittent positive pressure breathing with isoproterenol (0.5 ml 1:200) 15 minutes every hour may be necessary. Oxygen (6 to 12 liters/min) by mask or open top tent is essential. A short course of corticosteroid therapy is usually indicated after severe attacks.

Status asthmaticus. This connotes a condition of continuous severe asthma that is unrelieved by epinephrine or isoproterenol; it can be a life-threatening emergency. Failure to respond to beta adrenergic drugs may be due to a number of causes—such as obstruction because of mucosal edema or accumulation of viscid mucus plugs. Oxygen, mechanical ventilation, and ample hydration are administered as in any severe asthma episode. Aminophylline may be useful but should not be administered in a dosage greater than 0.5 gm/hr. Corticosteroids offer the greatest benefit, but their onset of action is slow. Hydrocortisone sodium succinate (Solu-Cortef), 100 mg, or methylprednisolone (Solu-Medrol), 80 mg, should be given intravenously and may be repeated every 30 to 60 minutes as needed. If epinephrine or isoproterenol is not demonstrably effective, it should be discontinued.

Overdosage of beta adrenergic agents may provoke severe disturbances in cardiac rate and rhythm. When the heart is hypoxic and hyperirritable, as is often the case with patients who require bronchodilators, dangerous cardioacceleration may ensue. Ectopic foci commonly arise in the ventricular network, precipitating first premature ventricular contractions (PVCs) and then, as their frequency increases, ventricular tachycardia which may progress to ventricular fibrillation. These serious complications must be treated by experienced clinicians. The presence of arrhythmia must be noted promptly; for this reason the patient with status asthmaticus should be treated in an intensive care unit with constant ECG monitoring. Ventricular fibrillation is immediately life threatening; it is the commonest form of circulatory arrest and requires the prompt application of electrical countershock (defibrillation).

REFERENCES

1. Alliott, R. J., et al.: Effects of salbutamol and isoprenaline/phenylephrine in reversible airways obstruction, Br. Med. J. **1:**539-542, 1972.
2. Amory, D. W., Burnham, S. C., and Cheney, F. W., Jr.: Comparison of the cardiopulmonary effects of subcutaneously administered epinephrine and terbutaline in patients with reversible airway obstruction, Chest **67:**279-286, 1975.
3. Aviado, D. M., and Carrillo, L. R.: Antiasthmatic action of corticosteroids; a review of the literature on their mechanism of action, J. Clin. Pharmacol. **10:**3-11, 1970.
4. Butcher, R.: Role of cyclic AMP in hormone actions, N. Engl. J. Med. **279:**1378-1384, 1968.
5. Chervinsky, P., and Herstoff, R.: IPPB therapy with bronkospray or isoproterenol—a comparison, J. Asthma Res. **4:**197-204, 1967.
6. Choo-Kang, Y. F. J., Simpson, W. T., and Grant, I. W. B.: Controlled com-

parison of the bronchodilator effects of three B-adrenergic stimulant drugs administered by inhalation to patients with asthma, Br. Med. J. **2:**287-289, 1969.

7. Clark, D. G., and Tinston, D. J.: Cardiac effects of isoproterenol, hypoxia, hypercapnia, and fluorocarbon propellants and their use in asthma inhalers, Ann. Allergy **30:**536-541, 1972.

8. Cohen, B. M.: Studies with isoetharine. I. The ventilatory effects of aerosol and oral forms, J. Asthma Res. **4:**209-218, 1967.

9. Cox, J. S. G., et al.: Disodium cromoglycate (Intal). In Harper, N. J., and Simmonds, A. B., editors: Advances in drug research, vol. 5, New York, 1970, Harper & Row, Publishers.

10. Gaddie, J., et al.: Aerosol beclomethasone dipropionate in chronic bronchial asthma, Lancet **1:**691-693, 1973.

11. Geddes, B. A., and Lefcoe, N. M.: Respiratory smooth muscle relaxing effect of commercial steroid preparations, Am. Rev. Respir. Dis. **107:**395-399, 1973.

12. Gould, L., and Dilieto, M.: Phentolamine, new bronchodilator, N.Y. Med. **70:**2332-2337, 1970.

13. Harris, L. H.: Effects of isoprenaline plus phenylephrine by pressurized aerosol on blood gases, ventilation, and perfusion in chronic obstructive lung disease, Br. Med. J. **4:**579-582, 1970.

14. Harris, W. S.: Toxic effects of aerosol propellants on the heart, Arch. Intern. Med. **131:**163-166, 1973.

15. Heurich, A., Sousa-Poza, M., and Lyons, H. A.: Bronchodilator effects of hydroxyzine hydrochloride, Respiration **29:**135-138, 1972.

16. Hodson, M. E., et al.: Beclomethasone dipropionate aerosol in asthma, Am. Rev. Respir. Dis. **110:**403-408, 1974.

17. Hyde, J. S.: Cromolyn prophylaxis for chronic asthma, Ann. Intern. Med. **78:**966, 1973.

18. Lands, A. M., et al.: Differentiation of receptor systems activated by sympathomimetic amines, Nature **214:**597-598, 1967.

19. Lewis, A. A. G., editor: Salbutamol, Proceedings of an international symposium, Postgrad. Med. J. **47**(supp.):1-133, 1971.

20. Lewis, R. A., et al.: Formation of slow-reacting substance of anaphylaxis in human lung tissue and cells before release, J. Exp. Med. **140:**1133-1145, 1974.

21. Middleton, E., Jr.: Autonomic imbalance in asthma with special reference to beta adrenergic blockade, Adv. Intern. Med. **181:**177-197, 1972.

22. Miller, W. F.: Fundamental principles of aerosol therapy, Respir. Care **17:**295-306, 1972.

23. Milne, J., et al.: Long-term study of disodium cromoglycate in treatment of severe extrinsic or intrinsic bronchial asthma in adults, Br. Med. J. **4:**383-388, 1972.

24. Nicholson, D. P., and Chick, T. W.: A re-evaluation of parenteral aminophylline, Am. Rev. Respir. Dis. **108:**241-247, 1973.

25. Orange, R. P., and Austin, K. F.: The immunological release of chemical mediators of immediate type hypersensitivity from human lung. In Amos, B., editor: Progress in immunology, vol. 1, New York, 1971, Academic Press, Inc., p. 173.

26. Orr, T. S. C., et al.: The effect of disodium cromoglycate on the release of histamine and degranulation of rat mast cells induced by compound 48/80, Life Sci. **10:**805-812, 1971.
27. Sackner, M. A., et al.: Bronchodilator effects of terbutaline and epinephrine in obstructive lung disease, Clin. Pharmacol. Ther. **16:**499-506, 1974.
28. Silverglade, A.: Cardiac toxicity of aerosol propellants, J.A.M.A. **222:**827-829, 1972.
29. Spector, S. L., and Farr, R. S.: Bronchial inhalation procedures in asthmatics, Med. Clin. North Am. **58:**71-84, 1974.
30. Storms, W. W., DoPico, G. A., and Reed, C. E.: Aerosol Sch 1000, an anticholinergic bronchodilator, Am. Rev. Respir. Dis. **111:**419-422, 1975.
31. Szentivanyi, A.: The beta adrenergic theory of the atopic abnormality in bronchial asthma, J. Allergy **42:**203-232, 1968.
32. Taylor, G. V., IV, and Harris, W. S.: Cardiac toxicity of aerosol propellants, J.A.M.A. **214:**81-85, 1970.
33. Townley, R. G.: Pharmacologic blocks to mediator release: clinical applications, Adv. Asthma-Allergy **2:**7-16, 1975.
34. Wilson, J.: Treatment or prevention of pulmonary cellular damage with pharmacologic doses of corticosteroid, Surg. Gynecol. Obstet. **134:**675-681, 1972.

3 Mucokinetic substances

Properties of bronchial mucus[7]

The tracheobronchial membrane is normally coated with a mucus blanket that is propelled from below upward by ciliary wave motion. The water content of this layer is probably derived from the cells of the bronchial mucosa. The mucus proper is elaborated by two types of secretory organs, the goblet cells of the epithelium and the bronchial glands.

In chronic bronchitis the goblet cells are markedly increased in number; they produce mucus that is more viscous than the product of the bronchial glands. Acute inflammation and allergic responses may cause production of profuse or tenacious secretions, and clearance may become a serious problem. This is particularly true if the patient is immobilized, debilitated by serious illness, dehydrated, or mechanically unable to cough. Respiratory failure in the patient with chronic lung disease most often follows an exacerbation of secretory activity, with mucus retention and consequent airway obstruction. Destructive changes in the lung parenchyma frequently accompany these episodes. The primary aim of therapy is removal of mucus, restoration of airway patency, and reduction of the work of breathing.

To understand the methods and procedures of bronchial clearance, one must have some knowledge of the properties of mucus.

The product of the goblet cell is a fibrous gel comprised of strands of mucoprotein in which aggregates of mucopolysaccharide are incorporated. Water and electrolytes are present in varying proportions, reflecting the existing volume and composition of extracellular fluid. Purulent sputum, which includes the debris of cell nuclei, contains fibers of deoxyribonucleic acid

(DNA) that increase viscosity, inhibit lysis of mucoproteins, and reduce the effectiveness of certain antibiotics. The presence of DNA confers a yellow color to mucus; and on standing the mucus becomes green. The viscosity of mucus is abnormally increased in mucoviscidosis and bronchiectasis. A common finding is an elevated calcium ion concentration in bronchial secretions. In alveolar proteinosis there is overproduction of a surfactant-like substance from the pneumocytes, and the result is a profuse viscid exudate.

Substances that promote dilution of secretions[4]

Dehydration is perhaps the commonest single cause of retention of secretions. Fever, failure of adequate intake, or gastrointestinal losses may so deplete the extracellular fluid stores that secretions assume the consistency of glue and plug formation is widespread. Bronchopulmonary infection or bronchial asthma may be seriously exacerbated if dehydration is allowed to occur. Medication with antihistamines or atropine-like drugs will impair secretory activity, and diuretics will contribute to fluid depletion. A particularly difficult problem may arise when chronic lung disease is accompanied by right heart failure, since circulating volume restriction is essential to restoration of cardiac function.

Water and electrolytes must be supplied in abundance to maintain mobility of profuse or viscid secretions. If oral intake is limited, intravenous supplementation is required. Nebulized water or ½ normal saline may be supplied by aerosol, preferably by ultrasonic nebulizer. Estimates of fluid intake by the inhalation route must be added to the patient's intake record. In the infant or small child, frequent weighing may be necessary.

The term *expectorant*, no longer current in pharmacology, signifies an oral preparation that promotes dilution or thinning of secretions. Generally it is strongly flavored and mildly irritating to the oropharynx; it is designed to increase the flow of extracellular fluid into the bronchial lumen. Gastric irritation and nausea are side actions commonly observed. The following is a list of compounds recommended for this purpose:

1. Ammonium chloride, 0.5 gm 3 times/day in liquid preparations
2. Sodium (or potassium) iodide, 0.3 gm 3 times/day, in saturated aqueous solution or syrup of hydriodic acid
3. Ipecac (as syrup), 0.1 to 0.5 ml every 3 hours
4. Glyceryl guaiacolate (Guaianesin), 100 to 200 mg every 3 hours[3]
5. Bromhexine (Bisolvon)[2] (available only in Europe)

Substances that alter surface tension

Certain hygroscopic chemicals (e.g., propylene glycol, glycerine) have been recommended as wetting agents and to stabilize droplets of nebulized solutions. Alevaire[1] and Tergemist were commercial preparations incorporating a detergent with other mucokinetic substances. Their use by inhalation is ineffective, and there is reason to suspect that such mixtures remove surfactant from alveolar surfaces. Ethyl alcohol, 20% to 50%, either nebulized or vaporized by bubbling oxygen through the liquid, is an effective antifoaming agent and has been recommended for treatment of pulmonary edema.

Substances that lyse secretions[5]

Two general categories of mucolytics exist: (1) those containing reactive sulfhydryl ($-SH$) groups and (2) proteolytic enzymes. The sulfhydryl moiety opens the disulfide bond of mucoprotein, reducing the viscosity of mucus:

$$2RSH + Pr-S-S-Pr \rightarrow RS-SR + 2Pr-SH$$

Acetylcysteine is the best known of the sulfhydryl derivatives. Others are dithioerythritol, methylcysteine, carboxymethylcysteine (Mucodyne), and 2-mercaptoethane sulfonate (Mistabron).[6]

Proteolytic enzymes are sparingly used, and only to lyse purulent secretions. Preparations include pancreatic dornase (Dornavac), trypsin (Tryptar), and streptokinase-streptodornase (Varidase).

Acetylcysteine (Mucomyst) is the acetyl derivative of the essential amino acid cysteine. It is rather unstable, requiring refrigeration, and it oxidizes rapidly on exposure to air. It is most effective when administered directly by bronchoscope or by bronchial lavage, in 10% solution. The pH of this solution is 7 to 9, the optimum range for mucolysis. Dilution greatly impairs activity; concentrations less than 1% are largely ineffective. Liquefaction of mucus is rapid, occurring almost immediately on contact. Recommended dosage for administration by aerosol is 6 to 10 ml of a 10% solution; when direct instillation is employed, 1 to 2 ml of 10% solution are sufficient.

Acetylcysteine is marketed in 20% solution, which is somewhat irritating and may on occasion require the simultaneous administration of a bronchodilator. This concentration is best avoided if possible since it is irritating. The sulfurous odor of both the 10% and the 20% solutions may be objectionable to some patients. Untoward effects reported include bronchospasm, hemoptysis, nausea, and vomiting. Acetylcysteine inactivates some antibiotics, particularly those of the penicillin group; these should not be administered in the same solution. Also acetylcysteine is decomposed by rubber or metallic equipment.

Pancreatic dornase (deoxyribonuclease) (Dornavac), as its name suggests, depolymerizes DNA. It is indicated only when secretions are purulent; the existence of pus cells or DNA fibers should be demonstrated before this drug is administered.

The dose by nebulization is 100,000 units of lyophilized enzyme dissolved in 2 ml of either normal saline or 10% propylene glycol, given 2 or 3 times/day for 2 to 4 days. The course may be repeated, but to give the enzyme continuously for more than a week is probably unwise. Pancreatic dornase is definitely irritating to all mucosal surfaces and may require an accompanying bronchodilator. Posterior pharyngeal soreness may develop; gargling with water after treatment should be routine. There are few clinical situations in which its administration by aerosol is indicated, and its use requires careful observation of the patient for reactions (fever, wheezing, dyspnea). Perhaps a more rational use is for external lavage of abscess cavities, such as those occurring in empyema.

Rational use of mucolytics[5]

To be effective, nebulized solutions must be absorbed from the mucous surfaces of airways. This frequently is a source of irritation and perhaps bronchospasm. Also there is the possibility of bacterial contamination. The best way to dilute secretions is to increase oral or parenteral fluid intake. The use of mucolytic substances is warranted only when simple addition of water to secretions is inadequate.

REFERENCES

1. Alevaire; notice of withdrawal of approval of new drug application, Fed. Reg. **38:**6305-6309, 1973.
2. Bromhexine (editorial), Lancet **1:**1058, 1971.
3. Hirsch, S. R., Viernes, P. F., and Kory, R. C.: The expectorant effect of glyceryl guaiacolate in patients with chronic bronchitis, Chest **63:**9-14, 1973.
4. Hirsch, S. R., Zastrow, J. E., and Kory, R. C.: Sputum liquefying agents: a comparative in vitro evaluation, J. Lab. Clin. Med. **74:**346-353, 1969.
5. Lieberman, J.: The appropriate use of mucolytic agents, Am. J. Med. **49:**1-4, 1970.
6. Steen, S. N., et al.: Clinical trial of 2-mercaptoethane sulfonic acid sodium salt in chronic bronchitis, J. Int. Res. Commun. System **1:**12-24, 1973.
7. Yeager, H., Jr.: Tracheobronchial secretions, Am. J. Med. **50:**493-509, 1971.

4 Muscle relaxants

For centuries the crude extracts of various plants have been employed by the South American Indians as arrow poisons. The term *curare* has been applied indiscriminately to these substances. The purified extract of one of these plants, *Chondrodendron tomentosum,* was introduced into clinical medicine as a muscle relaxant in 1942 and was soon succeeded by preparations of the pure alkaloid, *d*-tubocurarine.

To understand the intermediary effects of curare and related drugs, one must recall the fundamental physiology of the myoneural end organ.[1] Transmission of the nerve impulse to a muscle unit is mediated by the chemical transmitter acetylcholine. As the excitatory wave moves toward the muscle, this substance is liberated at the myoneural junction and promotes the depolarization of the so-called motor end plate of the myoneural unit. The result is a contractile response of the muscle fiber. The acetylcholine is almost immediately destroyed by a specific enzyme, acetylcholinesterase. The end plate becomes repolarized and the neuromuscular unit reverts to the resting state. It is then receptive to a new excitatory impulse.

Curare (*d*-tubocurarine), gallamine triethiodide (Flaxedil), and pancuronium (Pavulon) block or prevent the depolarization of the motor end plate by acetylcholine. They are categorized as *nondepolarizers*. Succinylcholine (Anectine, Sucostrin) promotes and then prolongs depolarization, thereby preventing response of the muscle to the following nerve impulses. It is called a persistent depolarizer or simply a depolarizer.

d-Tubocurarine preparations contain 3 mg/ml of solution, and doses of 3 to 10 ml are commonly required by adults. The intravenous route is practically always employed. Ordinarily the drug is administered in divided doses as the need for relaxation arises. Effects are noted within a minute, become maximal in 4 to 6 minutes, and usually disappear within 30 minutes. Small muscles (e.g., the extrinsic ocular group, muscles of facial expression) are most susceptible to the drug. Larger doses are required to paralyze the muscles of the jaw, abdomen, and extremities; the diaphragm is usually the last to be affected. Therefore, if the patient is apneic, a maximal effect has been obtained and further dosage will result only in prolonged curarization.

If proper ventilatory exchange is maintained, d-tubocurarine usually has little or no effect on cardiorespiratory function. Both oxygen supply and carbon dioxide removal must be kept within physiologic limits. A release of histamine is occasionally provoked and may result in bronchoconstriction or hypotension, especially in individuals with a history of allergy. Large doses injected rapidly intravenously may block transmission of autonomic ganglia. Marked vasodepression ensues, which may result in cardiovascular collapse. Sometimes this will occur at normal dose levels, particularly if other factors are contributory (e.g., low blood volume).

Gallamine (Flaxedil) is a synthetic nondepolarizing muscle relaxant. Its effects resemble those of d-tubocurarine, except that it is shorter acting (20 minutes or less). It is approximately one sixth as potent as d-tubocurarine; each milliliter of prepared solution contains 20 mg of the drug.

Gallamine does not cause significant histamine release; bronchospasm and anaphylactoid hypotension have not been reported. It exhibits an antivagal effect on the heart; tachycardia is usually observed.

Pancuronium (Pavulon) is a nondepolarizing muscle relaxant that is about five times as potent as d-tubocurarine. Its actions resemble those of curare, but histamine release is minimal. The solution contains 2 mg/ml, and doses of 2 to 3 ml are usually sufficient for 30 to 60 minutes of paralysis. Tachycardia due to antivagal action appears occasionally.[2]

Succinylcholine (Anectine, Sucostrin) is a closely related congener of acetylcholine; it is rapidly destroyed by cholinesterases and is shorter acting than the relaxants just described.

Succinylcholine is supplied in aqueous solution, containing 20 mg/ml, for intermittent dosage. Ordinarily 10 to 30 mg are injected to provide relaxation for short periods, as for intubation. The drug also is available in crystalline form, usually in 1 gm ampules that are added to stock intravenous solutions for administration by drip. The recommended concentration of drug in these infusions is 0.1% or 0.2% (i.e., one or two ampules/liter of fluid). The rate of administration necessary to provide adequate muscular relaxation varies widely among individuals; 2 to 3 mg/min is about average.

Reversal of nondepolarizing block

The actions of d-tubocurarine, gallamine, and pancuronium can be reversed to some degree by drugs that inhibit acetylcholinesterase—thus allowing an excess of acetylcholine to accumulate at the myoneural junction. These so-called anticholinesterases include neostigmine (Prostigmin), pyridostigmine (Regonol), and edrophonium (Tensilon). Neostigmine is most commonly employed, in intravenous doses of 1 to 5 mg, usually with atropine (0.6 mg) to suppress muscarinic side actions. The duration of effect may be no longer than 30 minutes, and paralysis may then recur. Thus in the presence of gross overcurarization, serial doses of reversal agent may be required or respiratory exchange may have to be maintained by mechanical ventilator until the overload of drug is eliminated.

Prolonged neuromuscular blockade

Muscle relaxants may be given for extended periods to facilitate control of respiration. This is of particular value in the patient requiring continuous mechanical ventilation who resists the machine. Muscle spasm or splinting, neurologic problems and mental confusion, hypoxemia, and tachypnea are frequent causative factors. The tachypneic patient may need to be controlled to prevent respiratory alkalosis. If not already obtunded, he should be well sedated before being paralyzed. Serial doses of d-tubocurarine (9 to 12 mg) or pancuronium (1 to 2 mg) are administered intravenously to sustain blockade. The procedure is useful in the management of head injury, flail chest, seizure disorders, and tetanus.

REFERENCES

1. Karczmar, A. G.: Neuromuscular pharmacology, Ann. Rev. Pharmacol. **7:**241-276, 1967.
2. Siker, E. S., Wolfson, B., and Schaner, P. J.: Muscle relaxants: advances in the last decade, Clin. Anesth. **3:**416-457, 1969.

5 Topical anesthetics

The performance of endotracheal intubation and bronchoscopy in respiratory care provides many occasions for topical anesthesia. Even insertion of a nasotracheal catheter may require a topical. The properties and particularly the toxic potentialities of local anesthetic drugs are of interest and importance when the therapist is involved in airway instrumentation.

Local anesthetics are drugs that interfere with nerve conduction; they are effective when applied to nerve roots, trunks, and filaments. It is essential that their action be completely reversible. Some of them penetrate the mucous membrane with facility and are useful for application to the upper airways.

Anesthesia of the nose, tongue, pharynx, glottis, and trachea can be accomplished by spraying a solution of the drug on the membrane. This is the most common method of administration but also presents the greatest risk of systemic toxicity.[1] Dispersal of the drug over a wide mucous surface with rich blood supply is followed by rapid absorption and escalation of blood level. A maximal effective concentration exists for each topical agent; increasing the concentration does not result in greater intensity or duration of action.[2] Overdose is largely preventable—by application of carefully measured volumes of solution with sufficient deliberation to prevent sudden rises in circulating levels.

Most local anesthetic drugs are vasodilator; cocaine is a notable exception. Occasionally vasoconstrictor substances are added to the solution to retard absorption, but these are of little value in topical anesthesia; systemic uptake and duration of blockade are essentially unaffected. Some shrinkage of the membrane results, however, and this may be of value in preventing epistaxis when nasotracheal intubation is performed. Phenylephrine, 0.25%, is recommended for this purpose.

Cocaine

Cocaine is an alkaloid obtained from the leaves of *Erythroxylon coca*, a tree indigenous to Bolivia and Peru. The discoverer of cocaine (Niemann, 1860) noted that it caused a numbing effect on the tongue. In 5% to 10% solution it produces anesthesia and intense local vasoconstriction, with blanching of the mucous membrane. Dosage should be limited to 2 to 4 ml. Cocaine is a potent central nervous system stimulant, which fact has led to its abuse and to restriction of its manufacture and sale. This objectionable property has detracted from the value of the drug, and consequently it has largely been superseded by its synthetic congeners.

Lidocaine

Probably the most widely used topical anesthetic at present, lidocaine (Xylocaine) is effective in 2% to 4% solutions. Dosage should not exceed 200 mg. The drug is also available as a 2% water-soluble jelly useful for application to endotracheal catheters and tubes.

Tetracaine

Tetracaine (Pontocaine) is available in 1% to 2% solutions. Its toxicity is much greater than that of lidocaine; the total dose should not be more than 80 mg. Its onset of action is slower but considerably more prolonged than lidocaine's.

Toxicity of local anesthetics

Due largely to arteriolar dilatation, rapid systemic absorption of lidocaine or tetracaine produces hypotension. Symptoms are those related to cerebral hypoperfusion; the patient complains of faintness, visual disturbances, vertigo, and nausea. Loss of consciousness may follow, which may be ameliorated by placing the patient in a recumbent position and administering oxygen. Prompt intravenous injection of a vasopressor drug may be necessary; and such a drug should be immediately available when a local anesthetic is to be given. Rarely cardiovascular collapse and arrest may occur suddenly, perhaps due to blockade of the cardiac conduction system. The depressant effect on conduction is therapeutically useful when dosage is carefully controlled. Lidocaine is frequently administered intravenously for prevention and treatment of arrhythmias, particularly those of ventricular origin.

All local anesthetics are stimulatory to the central nervous system. Agitation, restlessness, and tremor are early signs; convulsions may eventually ensue. Oxygen[3] and artificial ventilation are necessary and should be available at once. Seizure activity can be controlled with rapid-acting anticonvulsants, of which thiopental and diazepam[4] are most often selected. If the patient is obtunded, a muscle relaxant drug may be preferable. The stimulatory phase may be followed by depression, with respiratory and circulatory failure of central origin. Vigorous supportive measures, including intubation and continuous mechanical ventilation, may then be required.

REFERENCES
1. Adriani, J., and Campbell, B.: Fatalities following topical application of local anesthetics to mucous membranes, J.A.M.A. **162:**1527-1530, 1956.
2. Adriani, J., et al.: The comparative potency and effectiveness of topical anesthetics in man, Clin. Pharmacol. Ther. **5:**49-62, 1964.
3. Moore, D. C., and Bridenbaugh, L. D.: Oxygen: the antidote for systemic toxic reactions from local anesthetic drugs, J.A.M.A. **174:**842-847, 1960.
4. Munson, E. S., and Wagman, I. H.: Diazepam treatment of local anesthetic-induced seizures, Anesthesiology **37:**523-528, 1972.

6 Drugs affecting central respiratory centers

Sedation, hypnosis, and anesthesia (Table 6-1)

Drugs employed for sedation or to produce sleep comprise several classes of compounds. All are characterized by dose-related degrees of central depression, from a mild calming effect to deep anesthesia. Nearly all have been tried as anesthetic agents, and their actions at profound levels of depression are well known. Some of them, particularly the barbiturates, are commonly ingested with suicidal intent.

Virtually all sedative-hypnotic agents depress the entire central nervous system—including cortex, subcortex, midbrain, and medulla. The sleep-producing activity is correlated with depression of the central gray core of the brain stem (ascending reticular activating system). Presumably this is the portion of the brain concerned with awareness of external stimuli. Medullary depression is manifested at all dose levels. Depression of respiration is demonstrable at light levels and may be profound when the patient is deeply obtunded.

Much of the therapy of hypnotic drug depression is directed toward the restoration of adequate ventilation.[10,12]

Similarly depression of the vasomotor centers of the hypothalamus and brain stem results in a fall of blood pressure due to reduction of peripheral vascular tone. Treatment of drug overdose will often involve replenishment of body fluids and administration of vasopressor drugs to restore circulatory function.

An additional central depressant property usually seen among all classes of sedative-hypnotic compounds is anticonvulsant ac-

Table 6-1. Sedation, hypnosis, and anesthesia

	Dose (mg)	Duration of action (hr)
Barbiturates		
Phenobarbital (Luminal)	50-100	10-12
Amobarbital (Amytal)	100-200	6-8
Pentobarbital (Nembutal)	100-200	4-8
Secobarbital (Seconal)	100-200	4-6
Methohexital (Brevital)	25-50 (IV) initial	<½
Thiobarbiturates		
Thiopental (Pentothal)	50-100 (IV) initial	<½
Thiamylal (Surital)	50-100 (IV) initial	<½
Chloral hydrate	50-200	4-8
Piperidinediones		
Glutethimide (Doriden)	250-500	4-8
Methyprylon (Noludar)	100-300	4-8
Benzodiazepines		
Chlordiazepoxide (Librium)	10-20	8-24
Diazepam (Valium)	5-10	8-24
Flurazepam (Dalmane)	15-30	8-24
Hydroxyzine (Atarax, Vistaril)	25-50	4-12

tivity. This involves the suppression of a hyperirritable focus, usually in the motor cortex. Potent hypnotics, such as ultra–short-acting barbiturates, may be useful in controlling a generalized seizure. Other drugs, categorized as anticonvulsants, are often mild sedative-hypnotics with a potent suppressive effect on motor centers.

Table 6-1 lists the hypnotic drugs of widest current use, their average adult dose ranges, and their average periods of activity.

Barbiturates. These compounds are derivatives of malonyl-urea or barbituric acid. By suitable alteration of molecular structure, a large variation in onset, duration, and intensity of action can be obtained. All barbiturates produce sedation, hypnosis, and anesthesia with corresponding degrees of respiratory and circulatory depression. They can be divided into classes depending on their duration of action.

Long-acting barbiturates were the first to be introduced. They are stable in the body fluids, and a large portion is excreted unchanged. Their onset of action is slow (1 to 2 hours), and their effect persists for 24 to 36 hours. They are useful for continuous mild sedation, for control of moderate hypertension, and for suppression of epilepsy. Examples are barbital (Veronal) and phenobarbital (Luminal).

Intermediate-acting barbiturates are characterized by an onset of action of about 1 hour and duration of about 12 hours. They are useful for insomnia and anxiety states. Amobarbital (Amytal) is a representative example.

Short-acting barbiturates are characterized by a more rapid onset (20 to 30 minutes) and duration of about 6 hours. Brevity of action is due more to rapid distribution and sequestration of the drug in tissue depots, particularly fat, than to increased decomposition of the drug in the liver. Only about 25% of a typical short-acting barbiturate—e.g., pentobarbital (Nembutal) or secobarbital (Seconal)—is excreted unchanged. The remainder consists of breakdown products, some of which are unidentifiable.

Ultra–short-acting drugs are usually given intravenously. Their onset time is about 30 seconds, and the duration of a single dose is less than 30 minutes. They are used for intravenous anesthesia and as emergency anticonvulsants. Many of these drugs are derivatives of thiobarbituric acid, a closely related compound in which the oxygen of the urea residue is replaced by sulfur. Examples are thiopental (Pentothal) and thiamylal (Surital). A true barbiturate (oxybarbiturate) belonging to the ultra–short-acting class is methohexital (Brevital).

The patterns of barbiturate activity are related to the lipid solubility of the barbiturate, since this facilitates entry into cells. Thus a lipophilic compound would be rapidly distributed and absorbed and, in addition, would gain more rapid access to the liver microsomes (where the detoxication processes occur).

Barbiturates are poor analgesics and may evoke delirium in the presence of pain. They may also produce inebriation and must be employed with caution in aged patients and in drug habitués. Under ordinary circumstances, however, they provide satisfactory sedation and hypnosis; and they are useful in managing the anxious, restless, and apprehensive patient, such as one with respiratory insufficiency receiving mechanical ventilatory assistance.

Chloral hydrate. This compound produces sedation, hypnosis, or anesthesia according to the dose used. It is recommended for the elderly patient and provides a rapid relatively brief effect without inebriation or afterdepression. In the relatively small dosage usually employed (0.5 to 1 gm), respiratory and cardiovascular depression is minimal.

Piperidinediones. This group of sedative-hypnotics is chemically related to the barbiturates and is comparable to the short-acting group. The best known is glutethimide (Doriden); a similar derivative is methyprylon (Noludar).

Benzodiazepines. This class of compounds[7] includes diazepam (Valium), chlordiazepoxide (Librium), and flurazepam (Dalmane). These are relatively long-acting sedatives, usually free from marked side effects in therapeutic doses. Diazepam can be administered by injection, and intravenous doses of 5 to 10 ml are occasionally of value in acclimating a patient to the mechanical ventilator. Diazepam is also used as an emergency anticonvulsant.

Hydroxyzine. A large number of compounds of differing chemical structure possessing sedative-tranquilizer properties are termed *minor tranquilizers*. They are useful for the management of anxiety states. A few of them are particularly suitable in the management of patients on ventilators. Hydroxyzine (Atarax, Vistaril) is a minor tranquilizer obtainable in solution for injection which can be administered if needed to control the agitation and restlessness accompanying ventilator care.

Narcotics[9] (Table 6-2)

Crude opium has been known since the dawn of history and was prepared from the opium poppy by the ancients in the same manner as today. Morphine is its principal alkaloid and may be considered the prototype of the class of drugs known as narcotics. A rather specific group of effects is elicited by these compounds, some of which are of great therapeutic value.

Morphine. In therapeutic doses, morphine is remarkably analgesic and has long been employed for relief of severe pain. It can be assumed therefore to interfere with neuronal transmission in pain pathways, but this is difficult to demonstrate conclusively.

Table 6-2. Narcotics

	Dose (mg)	Uses
Morphine	10 ⎫	Analgesia, respiratory control
Hydromorphone (Dilaudid)	1.5 ⎬	
Oxymorphone (Numorphan)	1.5 ⎭	
Codeine	30-60 (10-30 antitussive)	Analgesia, cough
Hydrocodone (Hycodan)	5-10 (antitussive)	Cough
Oxycodone (Percodan)	10-15	Analgesia, cough
Dextromethorphan (Romilar)	15-30 (antitussive)	Cough
Meperidine (Demerol)	80-100	Analgesia
Alphaprodine (Nisentil)	40-60	Analgesia
Methadone	7.5-10	Analgesia, withdrawal syndrome
Fentanyl (Sublimaze)	0.05-0.1	Anesthesia, neuroleptanalgesia

Morphine produces depression of the central gray core of the brain stem, thereby diminishing overall awareness. It also produces euphoria in many patients, which doubtless contributes to pain relief. Morphine is markedly depressant to respiration,[5] a property of great usefulness in respiratory care. Even in small doses, the drug decreases the sensitivity of the brain stem respiratory centers to carbon dioxide, and this can be easily verified by experiment. The respiratory rate is markedly slowed, whereas depth is relatively unaffected except with an overdose. Thus the drug effect can be measured roughly by measurement of respiratory rate.

Patients with chronic pulmonary disease, flail chest, head trauma, or other conditions in which rapid respiratory rates lead to inefficient ventilation or exhaustion may respond favorably to morphine. To guarantee an adequate respiratory exchange, the drug must be given with the patient on the mechanical ventilator. Serial intravenous doses of 5 to 10 mg are usually effective.

Because of morphine's effect on the medullary vasomotor centers, some circulatory depression results. In addition, morphine is a stimulant to central parasympathetic (i.e., vagal) centers, producing bradycardia and smooth muscle spasm.

Parasympathetic effects include pupillary constriction, a common identifying sign in the addict that is reversed by hypoxia accompanying respiratory failure in drug overdose. Gastrointestinal stasis, producing constipation, is the result of spastic contraction of intestinal smooth muscle. Spasm also may occur in the biliary tract, the ureters, or most importantly the bronchiolar system. Bronchospasm, however, usually represents an allergic response to the drug.

Other important medullary effects of morphine involve the cough and vomiting reflexes. Morphine is one of the most potent antitussive (cough-relieving) drugs and must be used with caution if cough reflexes are to remain active. When control of cough is desired, a less potent narcotic (e.g., codeine) is preferable.

A medullary emetic center, the chemoreceptor trigger zone, is stimulated by morphine, causing vomiting in many individuals. Nausea may or may not be associated.

Finally, physical dependence on morphine is readily induced and withdrawal may result in serious illness. Unless the patient is already addicted, this dependence does not ordinarily become a problem unless drug administration is continued for more than 7 to 10 days.

Codeine. Another alkaloid closely similar chemically to morphine and present in smaller quantities in crude opium is codeine. It is much weaker than morphine, requiring a dose about six to ten times as great for the same analgesic effect. It is correspondingly less depressant to respiration and is less addictive. Although it has value as an analgesic and antitussive, it is of no value as a respiratory depressant for controlling ventilation.

Semisynthetic derivatives of morphine. Suitable alterations of the morphine molecule will produce narcotics that are more active than the natural alkaloid. These include heroin, which is approximately twice as effective an analgesic as morphine and is one of the most potent antitussives known; however, its extreme euphoria-producing activity has made necessary a law forbidding its manufacture and sale. Hydromorphone (Dilaudid) is a similar compound with about four times the potency of morphine. Although a natural alkaloid, codeine is more cheaply manufactured by the methylation of morphine. Several codeine derivatives

(hydrocodone, oxycodone) are available for treatment of cough.
Meperidine and congeners. Meperidine (Demerol) was for-
tuitously discovered in 1939; its narcotic properties were recognized, and its value as an analgesic soon firmly established. It is
about a tenth as potent as morphine, is not so euphorigenic, and
is less depressant to respiration. It is often favored when respiratory depression is to be avoided, such as after chest or upper
abdominal surgery. Also it is useful for obstetrical analgesia, to
minimize fetal depression. A congener of meperidine is alphaprodine (Nisentil).

Other potent narcotics. Methadone, discovered in 1941, has
approximately the same degree of analgesic potency and respiratory depressant effect as morphine. It is not so euphorigenic and
hence is not so addictive. It is useful for treatment of the withdrawal syndrome and is a highly effective antitussive.

Representative of another narcotic group is fentanyl (Sublimaze), which is 100 times as potent as morphine. It produces a
profound analgesia of short duration and is useful in anesthesia.

Many other molecular types have been discovered possessing
narcotic properties, some with high potency, as much as 1,000 to
1,500 times that of morphine. None of these latter compounds is
yet available clinically.

Attenuated narcotics. In many instances, pain relief can be
achieved without resorting to a highly potent drug. To expose the
patient to the hazards of respiratory and circulatory depression
and the risk of addiction would be unwarranted. Also it is convenient to prescribe a nonaddicting drug which can be obtained
without the restrictions of narcotic law.

One compound with attenuated narcotic action is propoxy-
phene (Darvon), a methadone-like derivative. Another is the
meperidine-like ethoheptazine (Zactane). Both have been marketed combined with aspirin to fortify their analgesic effects.

Antinarcotics

The observation by Pohl (1915) that N-allyl norcodeine prevented or abolished morphine-induced respiratory depression in
animals remained unnoticed for twenty-five years. Then, in

1942, Hart and McCawley discovered the more pronounced morphine antagonism of N-allyl normorphine, or nalorphine. This compound exemplifies a group of drugs that reverse respiratory and circulatory depression in narcotic overdose and precipitate withdrawal reaction in addicts. They possess analgesic properties, but to a lesser degree than narcotics. Also they may be dysphoric, or hallucinogenic.

Besides nalorphine (Nalline), levallorphan (Lorfan) and naloxone (Narcan)[8] are useful antinarcotics. Pentazocine (Talwin) is an analgesic with predominantly antinarcotic properties.

Tranquilizers and neuroleptics

Several groups of organic compounds suppress volitional activity, producing a state of apathy and reduced muscular movement. These are of value in the treatment of psychoses, particularly psychoses accompanied by agitated or maniacal behavior. Certain other responses characterize these drugs, among them antiemetic, hypotensive, and antihistaminic effects. Large doses frequently evoke reactions from the subcortical motor centers—the so-called dyskinesias, including muscular rigidity, tremors, the irresistible urge to move, and certain dystonic syndromes involving principally the face, neck, and tongue. Such undesirable actions can usually be relieved by drugs employed for the treatment of parkinsonism.

Rauwolfia alkaloids. These compounds, of which reserpine is the best known, were once employed as tranquilizers. Today their use is almost entirely confined to the treatment of hypertension.

Phenothiazines[6] (Table 6-3). An extremely broad spectrum of pharmacologic effects can be obtained from members of this class. Motor sedation, control of nausea and vomiting, antihistaminic, antipruritic (control of itching), and antitussive responses are obtainable with selected derivatives. All of them produce dose-related hypotension; also they may cause nonspecific changes in the electrocardiogram.[2]

Phenothiazines can be divided into two groups, those with moderate and those with high potency. The moderate-acting

Table 6-3. Phenothiazines*

	Dose (mg)	Uses
Chlorpromazine (Thorazine)	25-100	Tranquilizer
Promethazine (Phenergan)	25-50	Tranquilizer, antihistaminic
Prochlorperazine (Compazine)	10-30	Tranquilizer, antiemetic
Dimethoxanate (Clothera)	25-50	Antitussive
Pipezathate (Theratuss)	25-50	Antitussive

*These are only examples, knowledge of which is sufficient for respiratory therapists.

group is most frequently employed in respiratory care; the best known of these agents are chlorpromazine (Thorazine) and promethazine (Phenergan). A widely used representative of the high potency group is prochlorperazine (Compazine).

Butyrophenones. These are the most potent tranquilizers; their use is confined largely to situations requiring profound motor sedation. A special term, *neuroleptic,* is applied to a drug producing this marked state of depression.

Members of the butyrophenone class, such as haloperidol (Haldol) or droperidol (Inapsine), can be combined with potent narcotics for the production of anesthesia without complete loss of consciousness. The technique is termed *neuroleptanalgesia.*

Antitussives[4,13]

When cough is unproductive, racking, and exhausting, it may be desirable to obtund this important protective reflex. Phenothiazine derivatives employed as antitussives include dimethoxanate (Clothera) and pipezathate (Theratuss).

Nonnarcotic suppressives include benzonatate (Tessalon), which has local anesthetic activity, and carbapentane (Toclase), which resembles the antihistamines. Noscapine (narcotine, Nectadon), a nonnarcotic alkaloid of opium, has mild antitussive action and also relaxes bronchiolar smooth muscle.

Uses of central depressants in respiratory care

The principal indication for depressant drugs accompanying respiratory therapy procedures is the relief of anxiety and restlessness. A patient requiring intubation, tracheostomy, or positive pressure breathing for extended periods understandably will be apprehensive and may resort to irrational, hysterical behavior. Claustrophobia is a frequent response of these patients to the use of masks, shields, or tents. Simple reassurance may be inadequate unless fortified by a sedative. Since all central depressants may produce hypotension, particular care must be exercised to preserve blood pressure and protective circulatory reflexes. If the patient is breathing unassisted, depression of respiratory rate and volume should be avoided. Especially to be remembered is the fact that the hypoxia and hypercapnia accompanying hypoventilation are themselves depressant and may change a sedated patient to one who is deeply comatose.

Central depressants are of value to facilitate ventilator control. Usually the problem is tachypnea brought on by dyspnea, anxiety, or pain. A particularly common example is the patient with a crushed chest, in whom painful rib fractures and inefficient ventilatory effort combine to produce agitation and restlessness and a rapid respiratory rate. Narcotics given intravenously in small divided doses are often effective, providing the necessary analgesia and slowing of respiration to facilitate synchronization with the machine.

The patient on assisted ventilation with tidal volumes of 600 ml or more will often tend to develop a progressive respiratory alkalosis. It may be feasible to provide a moderate reduction in respiratory rate, which can be achieved by the judicious use of morphine or other narcotics.

Suppression of the highly irritable cough reflex usually requires a narcotic to depress the medullary cough center. Codeine and its congeners hydrocodone and oxycodone may be administered orally or parenterally; but more often they are simply added to a "cough mixture," a liquid preparation containing expectorants or nonnarcotic suppressives. An attenuated narcotic often used in these mixtures is dextromethorphan (Romilar).

Respiratory stimulants

Respiratory stimulation by drugs is seldom indicated. On occasion, however, a temporary improvement in ventilation will be effected by the use of a drug—thus obviating the necessity for mechanical ventilatory equipment. Pungent volatile substances (e.g., camphor, ammonia) produce reflex respiratory stimulation. Aromatic spirits of ammonia and ammonium carbonate (smelling salts) depend on the release of ammonia and consequent tracheobronchial irritation. The immediate efficacy of carbon dioxide as a respiratory stimulant depends to a considerable degree on local irritant action.

A number of central nervous system stimulants have been employed to activate the brain stem respiratory centers and thus augment ventilation. Although a long list of such drugs could be presented, only ethamivan (Emivan) and doxapram (Dopram, Stimulexin) are of current interest. These are convulsant drugs that can produce seizures by excitation of the cortical motor centers. In subconvulsant doses, however, they may provide sufficient brain stem stimulation to cause temporary increases in respiratory minute volume. Their use has been directed primarily toward the treatment of overdosage with central depressant drugs, particularly the barbiturates.

A few clinical reports have appeared in which a medullary stimulant was employed, as a "pharmacologic ventilator," for treatment of chronic respiratory insufficiency.[1] Improved oxygenation may be largely offset by the rise of oxygen consumption due to increased muscular activity, however, and unpleasant stimulatory side actions are frequent.[3] Doxapram has been used for short periods to avoid the need for mechanical ventilation when the underlying cause of respiratory failure can be rapidly reversed.[11]

REFERENCES

1. Bader, M. E., and Bader, R. A.: Respiratory stimulants in obstructive lung disease, Am. J. Med. **38:**165-171, 1965.
2. Ban, T. A., and St. Jean, A.: The effect of phenothiazines on the electrocardiogram, Can. Med. Assoc. J. **91:**537-540, 1964.
3. Bickerman, H. A., and Chusid, E. L.: The case against the use of respiratory stimulants, Chest **58:**53-56, 1970.
4. Bucher, K.: Pathophysiology and pharmacology of cough, Pharmacol. Rev. **10:**43-58, 1958.
5. Egbert, L., and Bendixen, H. H.: Effect of morphine on breathing pattern, J.A.M.A. **188:**485-488, 1964.
6. Forrest, I. S., Carr, C. J., and Usdin, E., editors: Phenothiazines and struc-

turally related drugs. In Advances in biochemical psychopharmacology, vol. 9, New York, 1974, Raven Press.

7. Garattini, S., Mussini, E., and Randall, L. O., editors: The benzodiazepines, New York, 1973, Raven Press.
8. Kallos, T., et al.: Interaction of the effects of naloxone and oxymorphone on human respiration, Anesthesiology **36:**278-285, 1972.
9. Lewis, J. W., Bentley, K. W., and Cowan, A.: Narcotic analgesics and antagonists, Ann. Rev. Pharmacol. **11:**241-270, 1971.
10. Mann, J. B., and Sandberg, D. H.: Therapy of sedative overdosage, Pediatr. Clin. North Am. **17:**617-628, 1970.
11. Moser, K. M., et al.: Respiratory stimulation with intravenous doxapram in respiratory failure, N. Engl. J. Med. **288:**427-431, 1973.
12. Robinson, R. R., Gunnells, J. C., Jr., and Clapp, J. R.: Treatment of acute barbiturate intoxication, Mod. Treat. **8:**561-579, 1971.
13. Salem, H., and Aviado, D. M., editors: Antitussive agents, In International encyclopedia of pharmacology and therapeutics, vols. 1 to 3, sect. 27, New York, 1970, Pergamon Press, Inc.

7 Oxygen

Almost from the time of its discovery (Priestley, 1772), oxygen has been recognized as important in the maintenance of life. Another hundred years were to elapse, however, before the toxic potentialities of oxygen excess were realized. The central nervous manifestations of high oxygen tensions were described by Paul Bert (1878); the deleterious effects on the lungs were identified by J. Lorraine Smith (1899). With the growth of our knowledge of anaerobic and aerobic metabolism, the biochemical role of oxygen has become more clearly defined. Although normal oxidative pathways are fairly well understood, our data concerning the aberrations caused by excess oxygen are still fragmentary. These changes may be best understood in the light of their manifestations on respiratory and cardiovascular functions.

To approach these topics, it is helpful to consider the properties of oxygen essential to life. For optimal maintenance of vital processes, about 250 to 300 ml must be absorbed into the arterial blood per minute; this requirement is increased as much as tenfold during exercise, fever, or hypermetabolic states. The deleterious effects of oxygen lack are widespread and will be reviewed briefly.

Hypoxia

Oxygen deprivation to tissue cells is soon manifested by dysfunction of organ systems leading eventually to irreversible injury and death. The oft quoted dictum of Haldane is apt: *Hypoxia not only stops the machine but wrecks the machinery.* Complete cessation of oxygen supply to the brain, as occurs in circulatory arrest, causes histologic changes in the cortical gray

57

matter in 3 to 4 minutes; these changes are irreversible after 5 or 6 minutes. The myocardium is also highly susceptible to oxygen lack since cardiac muscle cannot incur an oxygen debt. Renal and hepatic functions are seriously disturbed in hypoxic episodes.

Types. Evidently cellular oxidative processes will be curtailed if oxygen is insufficiently supplied or the cells are incapable of utilizing the oxygen delivered.

Etiologic classifications of hypoxia vary among authorities, but all are variations of Barcroft's four categories[3]: (1) *hypoxic,* inadequate saturation of hemoglobin, (2) *anemic,* inadequate functioning hemoglobin, (3) *stagnant,* failure of circulatory transport, and (4) *histotoxic,* impairment of cellular oxygen uptake. Perhaps as many as seven distinctive types can be differentiated:

1. Atmospheric. An ambient oxygen partial pressure of 100 torr must be provided. At altitudes above 12,000 feet, oxygen tensions fall below this; and at 33,000 feet even 100% oxygen fails to reach this value, requiring administration under increased pressure.

2. Ventilatory. Airway obstruction, underventilation due to restriction or muscle weakness, and ventilatory depression due to drugs, brain injury, or disease are the principal causes. Although oxygen therapy is unquestionably beneficial, definitive treatment must usually be directed to the etiologic factors.

3. Alveolocapillary. In this type, oxygen cannot diffuse through the membrane because of edema or infiltrative thickening; or an appreciable portion of venous return is not exposed to oxygen at all. The latter condition, termed *circulatory shunt,* follows lung consolidation in pneumonia. Venous admixture with arterial blood can also occur if there is communication between pulmonary and systemic circulations. The varieties of congenital cyanotic heart disease (e.g., interventricular septal defect) exemplify this. Oxygen is of value and will restore normal arterial content pending correction of the underlying condition—unless the proportion of shunted blood is too large (more than 20% of cardiac output).

4. Hemoglobic. Under normal conditions 95% of oxygen absorbed is transported in the circulation combined with hemoglobin. Reduction in total hemoglobin accompanying severe anemia or after exsanguinating hemorrhage may drastically reduce oxygen delivery. An identical situation occurs in carbon monoxide poisoning; the hemoglobin is inactivated by the formation of carboxyhemoglobin.

Some abnormal types of hemoglobin may combine readily with oxygen but will not release it easily at the Po_2 tensions found in tissue capillaries. In these rare instances, there may be inadequate tissue oxygen delivery in the face of normal arterial Po_2 values.

If large amounts of stored blood are administered, oxygen release may be impaired due to depletion of 2,3-diphosphoglycerate (DPG), an energy-rich metabolite found in erythrocytes that reduces the affinity of hemoglobin for oxygen. Thus, if oxygen tensions are within normal limits, tissue uptake may still be significantly diminished.[9]

5. Transport. Oxygen delivery to tissues is impaired during circulatory failure. The basic causes are insufficient circulating blood volume (hypovolemic shock), failure to maintain peripheral arteriolar tone (neurogenic shock), and congestive heart failure (cardiogenic shock). Other forms of shock may combine two or all three of these fundamental mechanisms.

6. Histotoxic. This is exemplified by cyanide poisoning, which inactivates the cytochrome oxidase system essential to cellular utilization of oxygen.

7. Demand. In hypermetabolic states (e.g., high temperature, hyperthyroidism) the tissue oxygen demand may exceed the supply. Then oxygen supplementation is essential.

Clinical manifestations. Interference with any of the oxygen-transport mechanisms, from ambient air to cell, produces the same clinical signs of tissue hypoxia. The symptoms are largely related to failure of brain function. Usually there is an initial phase of hyperirritability followed by depression. The patient with mild hypoxia is restless, garrulous, and emotionally labile; or he may merely complain of nausea or of being too warm. Reflex respiratory and circulatory stimulation produces air hunger and increased heart rate.

Cyanosis appears with marked desaturation; if the hemoglobin values are normal, it is seldom noted at an arterial Po_2 above 50 torr, representing 85% saturation. When the Po_2 falls to 40 torr (75% saturation), analgesia, apathy, and a loss of motor coordination are observed. Consciousness is lost when the Po_2 declines to 32 torr (65% saturation). At this point the myocardium begins to fail because of oxygen lack, further decreasing cerebral perfusion.

It should be realized that these symptoms appear only if the arterial Po_2 tension falls rapidly. Slow changes, as seen in patients with chronic lung disease, allow some adaptive mechanisms to occur (e.g., increased cardiac output and blood flow to the brain). In patients with chronic lung disease, the symptoms of hypoxia may occur only at very low Po_2 levels.

Although normal hemoglobin values are in the range of 14 to 15 gm/100 ml, the transport of oxygen is considered to be effective at somewhat lower values; however, hemoglobin concentrations below 8 to 10 gm/100 ml may be insufficient to support the patient under stress. A small fraction of the oxygen is carried in physical solution, and this can be increased by raising inspired oxygen tensions. Such a maneuver cannot increase the total oxygen content more than perhaps 10% to 15%; but, remember, dissolved oxygen is more readily utilized than hemoglobin-bound oxygen.

It must be emphasized that the primary indication for oxygen is *hypoxia,* in contradistinction to *dyspnea.* The hypoxic patient may not be dyspneic, and correction of hypoxia may not relieve dyspnea.

Effects of oxygen on vital functions

Perhaps the most clinically significant effect of oxygen at atmospheric pressure is respiratory depression. In normal man, 100% oxygen reduces respiratory minute volume 10%. This reduction is assumed to reflect the loss of chemoreceptor drive from the caroticoaortic area. Since respiration is normally regulated by the more sensitive mechanisms of carbon dioxide and hydrogen ion acting centrally, the effect of hyperoxia is insignificant when these reflexes are operative. When the brain stem sensors are depressed, respiratory minute volume becomes more dependent on the hypoxic drive of the caroticoaortic mechanism and the depressant effect of oxygen is greatly magnified. This phenomenon, usually termed *oxygen apnea,* appears under the following circumstances:

1. Brain stem depression due to drugs, brain injury, or disease
2. Progressive desensitization of respiratory centers by the elevated Pco_2 and depressed pH of chronic respiratory acidosis

Small decreases in cardiac output result when 100% oxygen is breathed. A mild bradycardia usually occurs, which is reversed by atropine and hence is considered to be vagal in origin. Due to improved myocardial oxygenation, the patient with congestive heart failure may show *increased* cardiac output. Moderate changes in peripheral vascular resistance are observed: in the systemic circuit there is a mild increase; in the pulmonary circuit a decrease is usually noted, especially after hypoxia.

*Pathologic effects on the lungs.** It is not surprising that oxygen toxicity is first manifested in the respiratory tract. Not only do the tracheobronchial mucosa and alveoli bear the initial brunt of local irritation, but the dilation of the pulmonic arterioles tends to aggravate the resulting hyperemia—a striking example of a compensatory mechanism functioning inappropriately.

Generally speaking, partial pressures of oxygen less than ½ atmosphere (380 torr) can be inhaled for several days with impunity. When the tension is raised to 600 torr, symptoms of respiratory irritation appear in about 12 hours: cough, sore throat, substernal distress, dyspnea. Animals exposed to 100% oxygen (760 torr ambient) die of bronchopneumonia in 2 to 8 days. The inflammatory process causes a marked interstitial pulmonary edema, accompanied by decreased compliance, atelectasis with rapidly developing circulatory shunt, and significant air trapping. At necropsy the lungs are heavy and the interstitium shows

*References 1, 2, 5, 7, 8, 13, 15, 16.

marked edema, lymphocytic infiltration, and fibrin deposition.

Pulmonary function studies on man receiving 100% oxygen reveal little or no change in respiratory parameters during the first 12 hours. Thereafter, the vital capacity steadily diminishes although the Pa_{O_2} does not fall appreciably until atelectasis is severe enough to cause a large venous admixture. It has been postulated that development of atelectasis parallels surfactant depletion. Recent determinations of alveolar surface tension indicate that this is essentially unaltered, even in the presence of advanced pulmonary changes.

The destructive process is accelerated by the presence of shock, severe hemorrhage, lung trauma, or irradiation. All these conditions favor the same alveolocapillary changes that have just been described. Prolonged periods of cardiopulmonary bypass, and even long-term hyperventilation with chronic respiratory alkalosis, predispose to early development of pneumonitis when high oxygen tensions are employed.

Corticosteroids afford no protection against the inflammatory responses of the lung; indeed, there is evidence that they augment tissue engorgement and development of atelectasis.

Central nervous system toxicity.[11] Exposure to high oxygen pressure (in excess of 2 atmospheres) produces marked sensory and motor dysfunction. A latent period occurs initially whose duration is inversely proportional to the oxygen tension. Symptoms and signs include twitching of the small muscles of the face and hands, cogwheel breathing due to diaphragmatic spasms, vertigo and tinnitus, nausea and vomiting, and numbness and paresthesias of the face and extremities. Myoclonic movements may progress rapidly to generalized convulsions. Usually the sensorium is clear up to the moment of onset of the seizure. If the oxygen is promptly diluted at this time, the individual recovers without sequelae.

The concomitant effects of carbon dioxide accumulation may be significant during administration of high oxygen tensions.[12] If oxygen apnea occurs, the cerebral complications are largely due to rapidly developing hypercapnia. These include cerebral venous engorgement and increased cerebrospinal fluid pressure, progressive narcosis, and eventually death from medullary failure. Muscular rigidity and tremors are frequently observed in hypercapnia, and carbon dioxide retention will decrease the seizure threshold to oxygen-induced convulsions.

Retrolental fibroplasia.[14] The systemic peripheral vasospasm induced by high oxygen tensions may produce retinal ischemia and fibrosis in the neonate, especially in the premature infant, whose retinal arteries are not fully developed. Exposure of these vessels to an arterial Po_2 in excess of 150 torr may cause irreversible obliterative changes with eventual blindness.

Evacuation of closed gas spaces. Administration of pure oxygen causes progressive nitrogen washout in the alveoli, middle ear, and paranasal sinuses. Subsequent absorption of the confined oxygen into the circulation may lower the pressures in these spaces to subatmospheric levels, resulting in atelectasis and pain in the ears and sinuses.

Cellular and biochemical effects of oxygen toxicity[4,6]

Many biochemical transformations occur in the absence of oxygen or in the presence of minimum oxygen consumption, as exemplified by the Embden-Meyerhof cycle. Much of embryonic development and the functional processes of muscular contraction, liver metabolism, and nerve conduction are anaerobic. When oxygen debt occurs, lactic acid accumulates; and the accumulating lactic acid promotes blood flow, suppresses bacterial growth, and stimulates vascularization. These processes are disturbed by a surfeit of oxygen, as the necropsy findings of oxygen-poisoned animals will attest. Cloudy swelling of most parenchymatous organs appears, and conductive tissues show edema and microsomal deterioration.

Aerobic processes are also deranged by oxygen excess. The biochemical mechanisms may be categorized as follows:
1. Formation of free radicals
2. Oxidation of enzymes
3. Depletion of inhibitory synaptic transmitter substances
4. Presence of oxyhemoglobin excess

Formation of free radicals. The oxygen atom contains six electrons in its outer shell, and it accepts two more in most of its chemical combinations; in other words, oxygen has a valence of

2. In this process of electron acceptance, there may be intermediate steps with the formation of electrically charged compounds known as free radicals. These are highly reactive and can disrupt biologic systems. Free radical formation is also promoted by ionizing radiation, and the cellular changes after roentgen ray exposure bear considerable resemblance to those following prolonged hyperoxia. The radiosensitivity of some malignant tumors can be enhanced by the simultaneous administration of hyperbaric oxygen.

Oxidation of enzymes. The action of a number of enzymes containing the sulfhydryl ($-SH$) group, enzymes that are essential to the cyclical oxidative processes, depends on the following transformation:

$$2RSH \underset{2[H]}{\overset{[O]}{\rightleftarrows}} RS - SR + H_2O$$

(active)   (inactive)

In the presence of oxygen excess, the reaction tends to move to the right, with formation of the inactive disulfide.

This is a special instance of a general transformation common to oxidative enzymes:

$$\text{Enzyme H}_2 \underset{2[H]}{\overset{[O]}{\rightleftarrows}} \text{Enzyme} + H_2O$$

(reduced form)   (oxidized form)

The effectiveness of these enzymes depends on the reversibility of the reaction. In the presence of hyperoxia, enzymes tend to persist in the oxidized form—thereby destroying their catalytic function. An example frequently cited is the disruptive effect of oxygen excess on nicotinamide adenine dinucleotide (NAD), an enzyme essential to several steps in the final common oxidative pathway, the citric acid cycle:

$$NADH_2 \underset{2[H]}{\overset{[O]}{\rightleftarrows}} NAD + H_2O$$

Depletion of inhibitory synaptic transmitter substances. The experimental observation has been made that the inhibitory transmitter in the central nervous system, gamma-aminobutyric acid (GABA) is depleted in hyperoxia. This is particularly true if convulsions have occurred. It is suspected that the oxidative biodegradation of GABA is accelerated by oxygen excess, thus releasing synaptic inhibition and promoting hyperirritability. The seizure threshold in animals can be raised by administration of GABA.

Oxyhemoglobin excess. An appreciable portion (about 20%) of the carbon dioxide returned from the tissues is carried in combination with hemoglobin. Reduced hemoglobin is more strongly basic than oxyhemoglobin and thus is a more efficient carbon dioxide carrier. In hyperoxia there is an excess of dissolved oxygen, which is preferentially utilized by the tissues; and much of the oxyhemoglobin is returned to the lungs unchanged. Hence, carbon dioxide transport is interfered with—resulting in tissue hypercapnia and the progressive development of acidosis. This deleterious process may be aggravated by the accompanying respiratory depression of hyperoxia, with consequent failure of carbon dioxide elimination.

Prevention of oxygen toxicity

In view of the profoundly disruptive potentialities of hyperoxia, it is axiomatic that oxygen should be administered at the lowest tension sufficient to maintain an adequate arterial Po_2 (i.e., 60 torr or above). Lambertsen[10] has stated that inspired tensions greater than 300 torr are poisonous. The concentration is apparently irrelevant; 100% oxygen at 250 torr is essentially nontoxic. Brain toxicity is encountered only at oxygen pressures above 2 atmospheres.

Oxygen cannot be stored in tissues for more than 1 or 2 minutes, and the milder effects of hyperoxia are quickly reversible. It would therefore seem rational to administer high tensions intermittently, if possible. The efficacy of cyclical oxygen therapy is confirmed by the clinical experience of many authorities, but this opinion is far from unanimous; and when high concentrations are necessary, they can seldom be curtailed even for brief periods.

If the patient is on continuous mechanical ventilatory assistance, microatelectasis may be prevented by periodic sighs or by administration of high tidal volumes. Often the necessity for high oxygen tensions can be alleviated by application of positive end-expiratory pressure (PEEP), which increases the area of alveolo-capillary membrane exposed and may improve oxygen diffusion.

Humidification. The irritant effects of oxygen are intensified by desiccation of the respiratory epithelium. It is essential that the gas be saturated with water vapor at body temperature when delivered to the patient. This can be accomplished by means of a heated humidifier, or by addition of nebulized water.

Administration. Safe administration of oxygen is predicated on the following principles:

1. Employment of as low a tension as possible to maintain an adequate arterial Po_2
2. Continuous administration of high tensions for no longer than 8 hours if possible
3. Periodic sighing to minimize atelectasis
4. Adequate humidification

Three general methods of administration are available: (1) nasal cannula, (2) face mask, and (3) tent or hood.

The *cannula* (nasal prongs) is the least uncomfortable and confining of the three. Concentrations of only 25% to 30% can be achieved at flows of 5 to 6 liters per minute, however.

Masks fitted with a reservoir bag are available to allow delivery of nearly 100% oxygen. This concentration is seldom required, however, and a more useful refinement is the Venturi mask—permitting a measurable air entrainment at specified oxygen flows. The Venturi mask is calibrated to deliver 24%, 28%, and 35% oxygen in currently available models.

Tents and *hoods* are now largely confined to pediatric practice. They lack the close oppressiveness of masks and cannulas but pose other problems, including elimination of leaks and maintenance of uniform temperature and humidification. For adequate control the oxygen concentration in the tent must be measured periodically with an analyzer.

REFERENCES

1. Balentine, J. D.: Pathologic effects of exposure to high oxygen tensions; a review, N. Engl. J. Med. **275**:1038-1040, 1966.
2. Barber, R. E., Lee, J., and Hamilton, W. K.: Oxygen toxicity in man, N. Engl. J. Med. **283**:1478-1484, 1970.

3. Barcroft, J.: The respiratory function of the blood, vol. 1 and 2, Cambridge, 1925, 1928, Cambridge University Press.
4. Chance, B., et al.: Intracellular oxidation-reduction states in vivo, Science **137:**499-508, 1962.
5. Clark, J. M., and Lambertsen, C. J. Pulmonary oxygen toxicity; a review, Pharmacol. Rev. **23:**37-133, 1971.
6. Cohen, P. J.: The metabolic function of oxygen and biochemical lesions of hypoxia, Anesthesiology **37:**148-177, 1972.
7. Haugaard, N.: Cellular mechanisms of oxygen toxicity, Physiol. Rev. **48:**311-373, 1968.
8. Joffe, N., and Simon, M.: Pulmonary oxygen toxicity in the adult, Radiology **93:**460-465, 1969.
9. Klocke, R. A.: Oxygen transport and 2,3-diphosphoglycerate (DPG), Chest **62:**79S-85S, 1972.
10. Lambertsen, C. J.: Effects of oxygen at high partial pressure. In Fenn, W. O., and Rahn, H., editors: Handbook of physiology, Respiration, vol. 2, sect. 3, Washington, D. C., 1965, American Physiological Society.
11. Lambertsen, C. J., et al.: Oxygen toxicity. Effects in man of oxygen inhalation at 1 and 3.5 atmospheres upon blood gas transport, cerebral circulation, and cerebral metabolism, J. Appl. Physiol. **5:**471-486, 1953.
12. Lambertsen, C. J., et al.: Oxygen toxicity. Arterial and internal jugular blood gas composition in man during inhalation of air, 100% O_2 and 2% CO_2 in O_2 at 3.5 atmospheres ambient pressure, J. Appl. Physiol. **8:**255-263, 1955.
13. Nash, G., Blennerhassett, J. B., and Pontoppidan, H.: Pulmonary lesions associated with oxygen therapy and artificial ventilation, N. Engl. J. Med. **276:**368-374, 1967.
14. Nichols, C. W., and Lambertsen, C. J. Effects of oxygen upon ophthalmic structures. In Lambertsen, C. J., editor: Underwater physiology, New York, 1971, Academic Press, Inc.
15. VanDeWater, J. M., et al.: Response of the lung to six to twelve hours of 100% inhalation in normal man, N. Engl. J. Med. **283:**621-626, 1970.
16. Winter, P. M., and Smith, G.: The toxicity of oxygen, Anesthesiology **37:**210-241, 1972.

8 Carbon dioxide and other therapeutic gases

Carbon dioxide[1]

Consideration of the pharmacologic properties of carbon dioxide entails a knowledge of the actions of the gas in concentrations exceeding physiologic limits.

When inhaled concentrations are less than 3%, the amplitude of respiratory movements is progressively increased as the fraction of inspired carbon dioxide (FI_{CO_2}) rises. Above 3%, carbon dioxide increases both the rate and the depth of respiration; at about 4% the respiratory minute volume (V_E) is doubled. At concentrations of 9% or 10%, the V_E is increased tenfold and respiratory response is maximal.

If inhaled concentrations are above 10%, carbon dioxide assumes the character of a central depressant—with progressive decrease of respiratory volume and vasomotor tone. At the same time, motor irritability is increased; convulsive seizures appear at concentrations of 20% to 30%. Respiratory exchange is abruptly decreased as convulsions appear. When concentrations are above 40%, there is rapid depression of brain stem centers, with respiratory and circulatory failure.

If carbon dioxide tensions are very slowly increased, the brain stem centers undergo a degree of compensation and densensitization. After a period of carbon dioxide breathing, the medullary centers become acclimatized to the point at which withdrawal of carbon dioxide will cause apnea. Ordinarily this will occur when the carbon dioxide tension has fallen about 5 torr.

Carbon dioxide promotes sympathoadrenal activation. The vasomotor centers are stimulated and circulating catecholamines are increased; stroke volume and cardiac output are augmented; and the heart rate is accelerated. Splanchnic constriction diverts blood to the coronary and cerebral vessels. As carbon dioxide tensions are further increased, the heart rate is slowed and blood pressure rises significantly. Carbon dioxide exerts a direct vasodilator effect on the peripheral vasculature. Flushing and sweating secondary to increased skin temperature are observed. One may notice increased oozing from cut surfaces in surgical incisions.

Sudden withdrawal of carbon dioxide excess may cause cardiovascular collapse due to abrupt central vasomotor depression. This condition is analogous to the desensitization of the respiratory centers just mentioned. Also the abrupt shift of pH to the alkaline side results in transmembrane shifts of potassium and calcium, which may increase cardiac and neuromuscular irritability. Ventricular tachyarrhythmias may appear and require immediate correction.

Even in low concentrations, the effects of carbon dioxide on the central nervous system are marked. Headache resulting from cerebral vasodilatation, nausea, and vomiting is common when inspired values are 3% to 5%. Stimulation of respiratory and vasomotor centers results in extreme dyspnea and palpitation. The individuals feels a sense of impending suffocation. A small but measurable degree of analgesia is demonstrable at this level. Concentrations of 10% to 15% produce marked apprehension, muscle twitchings, and considerable insensitivity to pain. Unconsciousness occurs after about 15 minutes of continuous administration. Concentrations of 20% to 25% produce surgical anesthesia, marked muscle rigidity, and eventual respiratory and vasomotor collapse.

A number of significant metabolic changes accompany continued carbon dioxide administration. Chief among these is progressive respiratory acidosis and a shift of hemoglobin dissociation favoring increased oxygen release (Bohr effect). Erythrocythemia occurs, and there is usually a marked decrease in clotting time. Blood viscosity is elevated. Due to increased glycogenolysis, blood glucose values rise—a typical sympathoadrenal response.

Carbon dioxide has few rational therapeutic uses. It may be employed cautiously to stimulate respiration in depressed states. The premature neonate with a tendency to apneic intervals may benefit from continuous administration of 0.5% to 1% concentrations. Some authors have maintained that carbon dioxide facilitates the metabolic breakdown of carbon monoxide hemoglobin and thus its use in conjunction with oxygen may be justified in cases of carbon monoxide poisoning. Respiratory alkalosis from hyperventilation may be rapidly corrected by a few breaths of 5% carbon dioxide in oxygen. The convulsant action of the gas has been utilized in shock therapy of schizophrenia, but this practice is no longer advocated.

Helium

Helium is an inert gas that is absorbed and eliminated from the body unchanged. Because of its very low density, it decreases airway resistance and diminishes the work of breathing. Since it is virtually insoluble in body fluids, total saturation and desaturation require about 5 to 7 hours. Diffusion time from an isolated lung lobule with circulation intact is about 26 hours.

Helium may be useful to facilitate respiratory exchange in cases of upper airway obstruction (e.g., laryngospasm, tracheal stenosis), since tracheal airflow is turbulent and resistance is a function of gas density. It is less useful in lower airway obstruction (e.g., asthma), where flow is largely laminar and therefore independent of gas density. Since helium (unlike nitrogen) does not produce narcosis at high pressures, it also can be used as a diluent for oxygen, to prevent oxygen toxicity, and to provide a safer mixture for deep-sea diving. Other clinical uses include its employment as a quenching agent in flammable anesthetic mixtures, as a carrier in gas chromatography, and as a contrast medium in pneumoencephalography. Helium is used in the pulmonary function laboratory for dilution tests to measure lung volumes and as a measure of gas dilution in determining carbon monoxide diffusing capacity. It is also employed to detect the effects of turbulence on airway conductance (iso–flow-volume curves).[2]

Nitrogen

Since man is immersed in a gaseous mixture containing 80% nitrogen, this gas is not ordinarily considered to have significant pharmacologic properties. It is biochemically inert and poorly soluble in body fluids. Diffusion from an isolated lung lobule requires about 18 hours, and desaturation about 6 to 7 hours. At several atmospheres pressure, nitrogen causes significant central nervous system depression. Drowsiness, failure of concentration, and inattention to safety measures have occurred in deep-sea divers from nitrogen narcosis. This is alleviated by replacing nitrogen with helium in the diver's tanks.

In addition to its use as an oxygen diluent, nitrogen has been employed as a quenching agent in flammable gas mixtures. In institutions where oxygen and nitrogen are stored in liquid form, compressed air has been reconstituted for administration to patients by appropriate mixing of these gases. Liquid nitrogen is employed for the rapid freezing of specimens of blood or other tissues and for cryotherapy (the destruction of tissue growths by freezing).

REFERENCES

1. Eckenhoff, J. E., editor: Carbon dioxide (symposium), Anesthesiology **21:**585-766, 1960.
2. Malo, J. L., and Leblanc, P.: Functional abnormalities in young asymptomatic smokers with special reference to flow volume curves breathing various gases, Am. Rev. Respir. Dis. **111:**623-629, 1975.

9 Antimicrobial therapy

General principles[9,17,18]

The therapist is seldom required to select the antibiotic regimen for a patient. This is such an important aspect of respiratory care, however, that familiarity with the common antibiotic and chemotherapeutic agents should be acquired. Also proper techniques should be learned when specimens for culture are obtained from the airway and from respiratory therapy equipment.[12]

In general, the organisms comprising the normal tracheobronchial flora become pathogenic only when host resistance is lowered. Most acute infections (e.g., those occurring in epidemics) are due to exogenous organisms. These are usually more readily controlled by antibiotics than are the organisms native to the upper airway. For example, the strains of *Pneumococcus* seen in lobar pneumonia are usually susceptible to penicillin in nontoxic dosage. Pneumonia caused by *Pseudomonas,* a normal inhabitant, is resistant to most antibiotics; and agents that control the organism are likely to be toxic at the dose levels required.

When antibiotics are to be administered, the causative organism of the disease process should be identified if possible. Cultures and sensitivity studies will usually indicate the drug of choice. These studies require a few days, however, and the patient's condition may not permit such a delay. Therefore, in the seriously ill patient the best guess is made by the physician and antibiotic therapy begun immediately pending the results from the laboratory.

In epidemics the offending organism may be correctly surmised. Infections in debilitated patients are likely to be mixed, and accurate bacteriologic appraisal is impossible without special studies. Under these circumstances a broad-spectrum antibiotic, to encompass as many of the likely pathogens is possible, is usually chosen.

The clinical response of the patient is an important guide to therapy. When prompt improvement is noted, the selected antibiotic may be assumed to be the proper one. If the infection is unchanged or progressive after 24 to 48 hours of treatment, the antibiotic is obviously not effective and a different one must be employed. Occasionally an effective antibiotic will have to be discontinued because of toxic side actions or an allergic response. The drug should always be given in adequate dosage since failure to control the pathogenic organisms may result in the development of resistant strains. Finally, when the therapeutic mission has been accomplished, the drug should be discontinued to avoid serious alterations in airway and gastrointestinal flora.

Failure of antimicrobial therapy may result from a lack of access of the drug to the site of infection. The pleural space is a familiar example. When collections of pus or foreign bodies are walled off by the inflammatory process, the circulation can no longer carry the antibiotics to these areas.

Mixed infections may require more than one antibiotic. Emergence of drug-resistant mutants may necessitate a change. As just noted, this may occur when antibiotic dosage is inadequate. Undue prolongation of treatment results in marked suppression of the patient's own organisms, particularly those in the colon, and may provoke invasion by organisms that are antibiotic resistant (a phenomenon termed *superinfection*).[20]

Adverse reactions to antibiotics

The basic principle of antimicrobial therapy is to utilize a drug with maximal toxicity to the pathogenic organisms but with minimal toxicity to the organs and tissues of the patient. Like all drugs, however, antibiotics have toxic side actions that may force their discontinuance. Since many antibiotics are themselves natural products, it is not surprising that allergic manifestations are frequently observed. Fever, skin rashes, and gastrointestinal upsets are the commonest allergic manifestations. A severe acute allergic reaction, termed *anaphylaxis,* is characterized by massive edema formation and circulatory collapse. Subglottic and bronchiolar mucosal swelling may cause fatal airway obstruction. These responses are due to the release of histamine and other products of tissue breakdown, which evoke widespread capillary dilation and edema formation with spasm of smooth muscle structures.

The allergic reaction may be delayed 5 to 10 days after administration of the drug. Urticaria (hives), fever, joint pains, and lymph node enlargement are characteristic and occasionally are termed the *serum sickness syndrome.* The syndrome may be confused with the patient's primary disease. Some hereditary predisposition to allergic susceptibility can be demonstrated. Also the patient with adrenal cortical failure is likely to show drug hypersensitivity.

Direct toxicity of antimicrobials is most frequently reflected by nausea, vomiting, and diarrhea. Some of the more potent drugs cause serious impairment of renal, hepatic, and hematopoietic functions. A few compounds, notably streptomycin, can damage the eighth cranial nerve (vestibulocochlear), producing disturbances in hearing and equilibrium.

As each drug is considered, its toxic potentialities will be noted.

Antibiotics

Antibiotics are specific chemical compounds derived from or produced by living organisms. In small amounts they can inhibit the life processes of other organisms.

Penicillin group. This comprises the antibiotics produced by *Penicillium notatum* and related species and their semisynthetic congeners. They possess the great virtue of being almost completely nontoxic in man. Allergic hypersensitivity is common, however. Anaphylactoid reactions may occur in sensitized individuals, with death from shock or airway edema. Every patient who is to receive pencillin should be questioned concerning previous reactions to drugs.

Except for some staphylococci that secrete penicillinase, the gram-positive bacteria are generally susceptible to penicillin. Penicillinase decomposes the antibiotic. Certain semisynthetic penicillins (methicillin, oxacillin, nafcillin) are unaffected by this enzyme and hence are useful for treatment of resistant staphylococcal infections. A few gram-negative organisms are sensitive to penicillin (*Meningococcus, Gonococcus*). Spirochetes (*Treponema pallidum*) are highly susceptible, and actinomycetes are relatively sensitive. Tubercle bacilli, most fungi, and all true viruses are penicillin resistant. Ampicillin (Polycillin) and carbenicillin (Pyopen) are active against many gram-negative organisms—including *Hemophilus influenzae, Escherichia coli, Klebsiella,* and some *Proteus* species. They are useful broad-spectrum antibiotics in mixed bacterial pneumonias. Diarrhea and skin rashes may accompany their use.

Antibiotics with activity similar to that of penicillin. The incidence of allergic response to penicillin approaches 20%. Therefore many patients are deprived of the usefulness of penicillin. Several classes of antibiotics possess similar spectra, however. Cephalosporins (cephalothin, cephaloridine,) derived from species of *Cephalosporium,* are closely related chemically to the penicillins. They are active against both gram-positive and gram-negative organisms, although usually not *Pseudomonas, Proteus,* or *Aerobacter.* They are relatively resistant to penicillinase and are often employed in staphylococcal infections. Erythromycin, lincomycin, and vancomycin are *Streptomyces* products that may be used in resistant staphylococcal infections.

Broad-spectrum antibiotics. This term is applied to antibiotics that are effective against both gram-positive and gram-negative infections and also against the larger subbacterial organisms such as the rickettsias. Ampicillin was mentioned in the discussion of penicillins.

The tetracyclines are represented by several closely related derivatives obtained from *Streptomyces* species. Tetracycline (Achromycin) is widely used for mixed bacterial infections, such as aspiration pneumonia. A compound with an extremely broad range of antibiotic activity is chloramphenicol (Chloromycetin). In influenzal meningitis, typhoid fever, and resistant staphylococcal infections, the action of chloramphenicol may be superior to that of other drugs. Cellular damage to the liver and bone marrow is a serious hazard, however, and limits the use of chloramphenicol to infections in which no other agent would suffice.

Streptomycin group. These are also known as the aminoglycosides, from their characteristic chemical structure. Streptomycin is effective against gram-positive and gram-negative organisms and against mycobacteria and spirochetes. It is employed effectively in tuberculosis and in severe gram-negative infections. Neomycin[4] and kanamycin[5] are often used against resistant *Proteus* and coliform infections or as a preoperative bowel preparation. Gentamicin is a relatively toxic drug; but it may be effective against certain gram-negative infections, particularly mixed pneumonias (including that due to *Pseudomonas*).

Streptomycin and congeners may produce toxic side actions involving the inner ear and kidney. Auditory and vestibular damage may appear after discontinuance of the drug and may progress after its withdrawal. Rifampin (Rifadin, Rimactane) is an unrelated antibiotic that has been substituted for streptomycin, particularly in drug-resistant cases of tuberculosis. Neomycin and kanamycin may cause renal damage and also are weak myoneural blocking agents. They may contribute to postoperative respiratory depression if muscle relaxants have been used.

Other antibiotics. A number of polypeptides, including bacitracin[14] and polymyxin B (Aerosporin),[16] are effective in many severe gram-negative infections but are likely to produce toxic side effects at therapeutic levels. Amphotericin B (Fungizone)[3,15] is employed for treatment of mycotic (fungal) infections. When these agents are used for treatment of pulmonary infections, their administration by aerosol has been recommended—on the theory that toxic systemic side effects may be diminished.

Chemotherapeutic agents

Chemotherapeutic agents are synthetic compounds that are usually simpler in chemical structure than antibiotics. They include the sulfonamides and sulfones, the antimalarial synthetics, amebicides, and anthelmintics. Many drugs employed in cancer chemotherapy also belong in this category.

Although largely superseded by antibiotics, the sulfonamides are still employed to advantage as anti-infectives. One derivative, sulfamethoxazole, is marketed in combination with trimethoprim, a drug akin to certain antimalarials.[19] The two drugs interfere with successive steps in the synthesis of essential nucleic acids and proteins by some bacteria; *Hemophilus, Proteus,* and *Klebsiella* species are susceptible. Trimethoprim-sulfamethoxazole (Bactrim, Septra) has been used for treatment of chronic bronchitis. It is also recommended for control of *Pneumocystis* infections of the lung. Another drug advocated for *Pneumocystis* pneumonia is pentamidine isethionate (Lomidine).[6]

A brief discussion of one of these groups, the tuberculostatic drugs, is pertinent. Isoniazid (Nydrazid, INH) is the best-known of a class of compounds that are potent tuberculostatic agents. It is a slow-acting drug and must be given over a period of months for full therapeutic effect. It also is a mild euphoriant, which property may result in undesirable hyperactivity of the patient. Toxicity is uncommon; but peripheral neuritis is occasionally seen and usually responds to administration of pyridoxine.

Aminosalicylic acid (Pamisyl, PAS) is moderately effective against the tubercle bacillus and exerts an additive effect with streptomycin or isoniazid. Ethambutol (Myambutol) is occasionally active against mycobacteria resistant to other drugs. Since the mode of antibacterial action is presumably different with each of these compounds, aminosalicylic acid and ethambutol are often used in combination with streptomycin or rifampin.

Administration of antibiotics by aerosol[10,11]

Control of bronchopulmonary infection cannot be achieved by topical application of an antimicrobial. Efficacy is dependent on an adequate antibiotic blood level, which is most readily reached by parenteral administration. The natural airway flora and inhaled microorganisms can to some extent be reduced either by direct instillation or inhalation of aerosolized solutions of appropriate agents. Serial doses of an antibiotic may be given via en-

Table 9-1. Antibiotics administered by aerosol (2 to 4 times daily)

	Dose (mg)	Reference
Carbenicillin	10-20	11
Gentamicin	40-120	13
Kanamycin	50-400	2, 5, 8
Neomycin	50-400	4
Chloramphenicol	100-400	11
Bacitracin	5,000-200,000 U.	14
Polymyxin B	10-50	16
Colistin	2-10	13
Amphotericin B	5-20	3, 15

dotracheal tube or through an indwelling transtracheal cathether.[1] The procedure is wasteful; dosage is imprecise; and if the drug is expensive, administration by this route may be unfeasible. The risks of untoward systemic effects of toxic antibiotics, however, are diminished. Efforts have been made to control infection in bronchiectasis and cystic fibrosis by preventing colonization of invasive organisms.

Carbenicillin is the only penicillin derivative that has been recommended. Gentamicin,[7,13] neomycin,[4] kanamycin,[2,8] and chloramphenicol are reported to be beneficial for control of gram-negative bronchial organisms. The toxic agents bacitracin,[14] polymyxin B,[16] colistin,[13] and amphotericin B[3,15] have been employed by aerosol; the last may provide an approach to treatment of fungal growths in the lung. Instilled via transtracheal catheter, amphotericin B is reported to be effective in resolving the granulomatous lesions of aspergillosis.

Table 9-1 summarizes some current opinions concerning antibiotics administered by aerosol.

REFERENCES

1. Aslam, P. A., et al.: Endocavitary infusion through percutaneous endobronchial catheter, Chest **57**:94-96, 1970.
2. Bilodeau, M., Roy, J. C., and Giroux, M.: Studies of absorption of kanamycin by aerosolization, Ann. N.Y. Acad. Sci. **132**:870-878, 1966.
3. Eisenberg, R. S., and Oatway, W. H.: Nebulization of amphotericin B, Am. Rev. Respir. Dis. **103**:289-292, 1971.
4. Gibbs, G. E., and Raskin, J.: Neomycin aerosol in the pulmonary complication of cystic fibrosis of the pancreas, Antibiot. Med. **2**:332-336, 1956.

5. High, R. H., Sarria, A., and Huang, N. N.: Kanamycin in the treatment of infections in infants and children, Ann. N.Y. Acad. Sci. **76:**289-307, 1958.
6. Ivady, G., et al.: Pneumocystis carinii pneumonia, Lancet **1:**616-617, 1967.
7. Klastersky, J., et al.: Endotracheal gentamicin in bronchial infection in patients with tracheostomy, Chest **61:**117-120, 1972.
8. Lifschitz, M. I., and Denning, C. R.: Safety of kanamycin aerosol, Clin. Pharmacol. Ther. **12:**91-95, 1971.
9. Macaraeg, P. V. J., Lasagna, L., and Bianchine, J. R. A study of hospital staff attitudes concerning the comparative merits of antibiotics, Clin. Pharmacol. Ther. **12:**1-12, 1971.
10. Miller, W. F.: Antibiotic aerosols. In Kagan, B. M., editor: Antimicrobial therapy, Philadelphia, 1970, W. B. Saunders Co.
11. Miller, W. F., and Johnston, F. F.: Use of ultrasonic aerosols with ventilatory assistors, J. Asthma Res. **5:**335-354, 1968.
12. Pierce, A. K., et al.: Long-term evaluation of decontamination of inhalation therapy equipment, N. Engl. J. Med. **282:**528-531, 1970.
13. Pines, A., Raafat, H., and Plucinski, K.: Gentamicin (Garamycin) and colistin in chronic purulent bronchial infections, Br. Med. J. **1:**543-545, 1967.
14. Prigal, S. J., and Furman, M. L.: The use of bacitracin, a new antibiotic, in aerosol form, Ann. Allergy **7:**662-675, 1949.
15. Ramirez, R. J.: Pulmonary aspergilloma: endobronchial treatment, N. Engl. J. Med. **271:**1281-1285, 1964.
16. Ramirez, R. J., and O'Neill, E. F.: Endobronchial polymyxin B: experimental observations in chronic bronchitis, Chest **58:**352-357, 1970.
17. Resztak, K. E., and Williams, R. B. A review of antibiotic therapy in patients with systemic infections, Am. J. Hosp. Pharm. **29:**935-941, 1972.
18. Roberts, A. W., and Visconti, J. A.: The rational and irrational use of systemic antimicrobial drugs, Am. J. Hosp. Pharm. **29:**828-834, 1972.
19. Trimethoprim-sulfamethoxazole (symposium), J. Infect. Dis. **128**(supp.): 425-816, 1973.
20. Weinstein, L.: Superinfection; a complication of antimicrobial therapy and prophylaxis, Am. J. Surg. **107:**704-709, 1964.

Glossary

aerosol A solution of a drug that can be atomized into a fine mist for respiratory therapy.

affinity Attraction for, tendency to combine with.

agonist A drug that combines with a receptor and initiates a pharmacologic effect.

allergy A hypersensitive state acquired through exposure to a particular substance termed an *allergen*.

anaphylaxis An exaggerated antigen-antibody reaction characterized by massive edema and shock.

antagonist A drug that opposes the action of a given agonist. It may combine with the same cell receptor but does not trigger the pharmacologic effect of the agonist.

antibiotic A chemical substance produced by microorganisms which can, in dilute solutions, destroy bacteria or other microorganisms.

antibody A protein substance synthesized by the body in response to a stimulus, usually another substance termed an antigen.

antigen A foreign substance that when introduced into the body stimulates the formation of a specific antagonist termed an *antibody*.

dose The proper quantity of a drug to be administered at a given time.

efficacy The therapeutic effect attainable by a drug.

idiosyncrasy Excessive or abnormal response to ordinary doses of a drug.

isomers Chemical compounds with the same percentage composition of elements but different molecular structures.

mucolytic Destroying or dissolving mucus.

parenteral Not through the alimentary canal, by injection.

placebo An inactive drug or preparation whose therapeutic effect is solely the result of suggestion.

receptor A chemical group or configuration on a cell surface capable of combining with a drug molecule.

resistance Reduced responsiveness to a drug.

sensitivity Increased responsiveness to a drug.

side effect A drug action other than the therapeutic effect.

specificity The degree of individuality shown by a drug in its union with the receptor.

stereoisomers Isomers (q.v.) whose differences are demonstrable only by three-dimensional representations.

synergism The combined effect of drugs, which is greater than the algebraic sum of their individual effects.

tachyphylaxis Rapidly decreasing responses after consecutive administrations of a drug.

therapeutic index The ratio of the lethal dose to the therapeutic dose of a drug.

tolerance Diminishing pharmacologic response to a drug on repeated administration.

topical Externally applied to the skin or mucous membrane.

Index

A

Aarane for bronchial asthma, 28
Acetylcholine in mediation of ganglionic transmission, 12
Acetylcysteine as mucolytic, 35-36
Achromycin as broad-spectrum antibiotic, 75
Adenosine monophosphate conversion to adenosine triphosphate, 16-17
Adenosine triphosphate, conversion of adenosine monophosphate to, 16-17
Adenylate cyclase in catalyzation of cyclic AMP formation, 17
Administration of drugs, routes of, 1-3
Adrenaline, 19, 22
Adrenergic compounds, beta, 23-24
Adrenergic drugs, 13, 18-24
Adrenolytic drugs, 14
Aerosolized bronchodilators
    clinical use of, 24-28
    recommended doses of, 22
Aerosols
    administration of antibiotics by, 77-78
    pressurized, dangers from, 24
Aerosporin for gram-negative infections, 76
Agonist, definition of, 5, 7
Alevaire, effect of, on surface tension of bronchial secretions, 35
Alkaloids, *Rauwolfia,* 52
Allergic reactions to antibiotics, 73-74
Allergy to drugs, 9
Alpha adrenergic drugs, 13
Alpha adrenolytic drugs, 25
Alpha receptors, drugs acting primarily on, 18-19
Alphaprodine, 51
Alveolocapillary hypoxia, 58
Aminoglycosides, 76

Metabolic effects of carbon dioxide, 69
Metaproterenol, 23, 24
    nebulized, for acute asthma, 29
Methacholine, reaction of asthmatics to, 18
Methadone, actions and uses of, 51
Methohexital as ultra–short-acting barbiturate, 46, 47
Methoxyphenamine, 24
Methylcysteine as mucolytic, 35
Methylprednisolone for status asthmaticus, 30
Methylxanthines, 25-26
Methyprylon as sedative-hypnotic, 48
Mistabron as mucolytic, 35
Morphine, 48-50
    semisynthetic derivatives of, 50-51
Motor systems
    drugs affecting, 14
    as site of action of drugs, 10-12
Mucodyne as mucolytic, 35
Mucokinetic substances, 33-37
Mucolytics, rational use of, 37
Mucomyst as mucolytic, 35-36
Mucus, bronchial, properties of, 33-34
Muscarinic actions of acetylcholine, 12
Muscle relaxants, 38-41
Myambutol for mycobacteria, 77
Myoneural blocking agents, 13

N

Nalline as morphine antagonist, 52
N-Allyl normorphine as morphine antagonist, 52
Nalorphine as morphine antagonist, 52
Naloxone as antinarcotic, 52
Narcan as antinarcotic, 52
Narcotics, 48-51
    attenuated, 51
Narcotine as antitussive, 53
Nectadon as antitussive, 53
Nembutal as short-acting barbiturate, 46, 47
Neomycin
    for gram-negative bronchial organisms, 78
    uses and side effects of, 76
Neostigmine for reversal of nondepolarizing block, 40
Neuroleptanalgesia, drugs used for, 53
Neuroleptics, 52-53
Neuromuscular blockade, prolonged, 40-41

S

Secobarbital as short-acting barbiturate, 46, 47
Seconal as short-acting barbiturate, 46, 47
Secretions, bronchial
    properties of, 33-34
    substances lysing, 35-36
    substances promoting dilution of, 34-35
    surface tension of, substances altering, 35
Sedation, drugs producing, 45-48
Septra, uses of, 77
Serum sickness syndrome, 74
Solu-Cortef for status asthmaticus, 30
Somatic system, physiology of, 10-11
Status asthmaticus, 29-30
Stimulants, respiratory, 54-55
Stimulexin as respiratory stimulant, 55
Streptokinase-streptodornase as mucolytic, 35
Streptomycin group of antibiotics, 76
Structure-activity relations of drugs, 4-8
Sublimaze, use of, 51
Succinylcholine as muscle relaxant, 38, 39-40
Sucostrin as muscle relaxant, 38, 39-40
Sudafed as oral decongestant, 23
Sulfhydryl, mucolytics containing, 35
Sulfonamides as anti-infectives, 77
Superinfection, definition of, 8, 73
Surface tension of bronchial secretions, substances altering, 35
Surital as ultra–short-acting barbiturate, 46, 47
Sympathetic division of autonomic system, physiology of, 11-12
Synergism, drug, 9

T

Talwin as analgesic, 52
Tensilon for reversal of nondepolarizing block, 40
Tension, surface, of bronchial secretions, substances altering, 35
Tents for oxygen administration, 66
Terbutaline, 23
Tergemist, effect of, on surface tension of bronchial secretions, 35
Tessalon as antitussive, 53
Tetracaine, 43
Tetracyclines as broad-spectrum antibiotics, 75
Theophylline ethylenediamine, 26
Therapeutic index, 8
Therapeutics, definition of, 1
Theratuss as antitussive, 53